Acknowledgement

A big thank you to all my friends and family who contributed recipes and have supported me and to my work colleagues who have had to put up my ranting about health benefits of certain food each time I did a new piece of research. And a special thank you to my long suffering husband who has had to sample all the new quirky foods I have researched.

About the author.

I am a forty something foodie who has tried almost every diet ever with the result of losing then regaining my excess weight and feeling rotten about it.
I realised that my short term goals were failing so I thought to try a long term strategy. I lose a few pounds a month with minimal effort and my skin, hair and general health have never been better.
I enjoy a few drinks –probably too many – I enjoy good food and good company and still maintain a steady weight loss.
I have found a way to feel healthier and lose weight without restricting my enjoyment of life.
I love it
I hope you do too.

Contents

Welcome

If you have picked up this book you have taken the first step towards gaining and retaining your ideal body weight and size. It's not about losing weight quickly and in the short term it's about understanding a little about how your body works and working with it to get an intelligent relationship with food. Getting to your ideal weight and size is not about perfection, it is about persistence.

You will slip up but that is just because you are human and not very perfect. If you had no issues with food and weight you would not be reading this.

The ideas in this book worked for me and they are going to work on getting you to that ideal you and in a way that is sustainable and not too much like hard work.

It won't be super quick but it will be a lasting and permanent change in the way you relate to food and eating, the way you think about food and the way you curb the urge to splurge. Your aim is to reach a stage when you are thinking about food only when you are actually hungry and when you are eating, savouring every mouthful. Maybe even eating a bit better and more mindfully but definitely not dieting.

So many people put off a diet until after a special occasion maybe a holiday or party because a diet will require deprivation of some sort.
A diet is a restriction.
A diet is not fun.

This is not a diet
The beauty of this system is that you don't have to wait until after Christmas or holiday – you can start right now.
'The diet starts tomorrow' is a familiar expression.
This is not a diet
Start now.
Today. Any minute.

Remember – **Persistence not perfection**
To get started you just have to follow Six Simple Rules

The Rules Bit

First Rule

No goals and no time limits

You cannot rush sustainable weight loss.

If you try to rush, you will fail. My definition of rushing is to undertake any attempt at obtaining a specific goal in any timescale.

Historically I can almost guarantee you have set short term goals - maybe aiming at a specific event – and used a short term strategy to achieve your goal. Short term goals encourage short term thinking.
In the short term this may have worked but if it were sustainable you would not be reading this now so let go of the urge to rush into your new eating habits.
But everybody knows goals are motivating, don't they? Well if they were motivating for weight loss we would all be successfully sustaining our ideal body shape and size? Setting a goal seems almost like setting a date to start the next unsuccessful attempt to stay trim once the current one has failed.
When it comes to losing weight and feeling fitter goals simply set you up to feel like a failure every time you make an unwise food choice. Stop beating yourself up – you will make poor choices but if you aim at a long term strategy the overall result will not be affected. It took you a long time to gain the weight you have; it will take a long time to lose it. This is a good thing. Long slow weight loss will last.
Even if you only lose one pound a week and then put half a pound back on that still equates to nearly two stone in a year. Over that space of time you will have changed your eating habits sufficiently to sustain that loss. If you don't put the half a pound back on you will have achieved a loss of three and a half

stone. I am not suggesting that you set a goal of a year – just using it to illustrate your potential.

If you don't want to diet you don't set goals and you don't limit yourself with deadlines.

Second Rule

For the next few weeks note what you eat and when

If you are eating unconsciously how can you consciously stop?

Ever seen that secret eater TV program? If not, tune in at least once.
I started to note down everything that I consumed, including tasting when I was cooking. I was very surprised. I thought I consumed a reasonable amount of food and always attributed my weight gain my love of wine and cider. I was surprised at how many little nibbles happened unconsciously during the day. If there is one absolute step that will help you – keeping a food notebook will do it. It will make you think about what you eat, when you eat and it helps to ask why that food and at that time. Even thinking about your emotions when eating could help you understand your food triggers. I know it sounds like a pain but it is statistically proven that if you keep a food diary you will lose more weight than if you do not. It will help further down the line when you take a baby step towards changing your relationship with food.
Keep it simple but keep it updated. If you want to lose weight you will ignore that internal chat that tells you it is too much like hard work, tell it to shut up and spend a couple of weeks looking closely at what you are eating.

If you don't want to diet – you need to understand why you eat what you eat and when.

Third Rule

Eat when you are hungry.

Hunger is there for a reason. It is your body's way of letting you know it needs something. One thing to learn how to distinguish physical hunger from emotional hunger.
Real hunger builds slowly as you body realises its need to replenish its energy levels and nutrients.
Emotional hunger is fast and furious and suddenly there.
Emotional hunger can be overcome it by various techniques – try to resist this sudden urge to eat unless you are really hungry.
Hunger is not always bad. This sounds nuts but it is a whole bunch of feelings and sensations. Try enjoying it once in a while.

Genuine hunger can sometimes be confused with thirst so try a glass of water – if still hungry – EAT.

If you don't want to diet you need to listen to and understand your body's needs.

Fourth Rule

Eat Slowly

Really slowly
Chew properly
Enjoy the textures
The flavours

That's not really why you are doing it – your body will start to send you signals when it is beginning to feel sated. It takes a little while for these signals to reach your brain and also for you to realise that this is what is happening. (About twenty minutes actually) This idea has been around forever but we never really take any notice of it.
From now on you are going to try to listen to your body. When it is telling you that you are really hungry – you double check to make sure it is real hunger – then you eat. Then you listen until it gives you the signs to let you know you have eaten enough.

If you don't want to diet you need to learn to listen out for the signals that tell us you have eaten enough.

Fifth Rule

When you have eaten enough – STOP

Sounds easy? It is much easier if you have followed rule four. Once your clever old body tells you it is satisfied it is time to put down the knife, fork, spoon or chopsticks and enjoy that sated feeling. Not the bloated to the point of exploding feeling – just pleasantly satisfied.
Resign from the clean plate club. Cleaning your plate is not helping anyone.
Waste is better than waist.
Eventually you will learn to reduce your portion sizes in line with your genuine appetite. Maybe try to reduce the portions immediately, maybe by about five percent. After all you can always have more but the temptation to clear your plate is very strong and usually instilled in childhood. But you are not a child so tell your inner kiddo that there is no one to tell you off for leaving a bit on your plate. I challenge you to leave a little something on every plate for the next month.

If you don't want to diet you need to learn to stop when you have had enough.

Sixth Rule

Keep Going – Persistence not perfection

Had a bad day at work? Keep going
Row with partner? Not an excuse to give up.
Slipped up? Accidentally ate an elephant? – Get back on track.

The only way you can fail is to stop
You will screw up but that's no excuse to stop.
This is your life, your body, your time and your choice.
And it is not a diet so what's to give up on?

If you don't want to diet you just have to be persistent in the little changes that mean you never have to diet again.

The Handy Hints Bit

Those are the rules – here are the handy hints

1. Weigh yourself as often as you like and get used to your weight going up and down. After a while the novelty and disappointment wears off. You will gain and lose weight but in the long term you will lose weight.
2. Remove temptation where possible to avoid unconscious eating. A packet of biscuits on your desk is asking for trouble. Out of sight is out of mind.
3. Eat breakfast every day. Don't skip it unless you are genuinely not even slightly hungry. If you can't face food have tea, coffee or lemon juice in hot water. Even just a piece of fruit is better than nothing at all.
4. Don't 'should' on yourself. If you don't do what you should do – forgive yourself. Every poor choice is a good opportunity to get back on with better choices.
5. Remove or reduce one thing from your usual food choices. Make two cookies just one cookie see if you really notice the difference. Change from sugar to stevia. Something small and simple. If you don't like the change, change back but try it, maybe.
6. Always leave something on your plate
7. Don't eat because it is time to eat – eat when you are hungry, only when you are hungry.
8. Don't eat because you are afraid you will offend your host. Likewise don't clear your plate from politeness
9. Don't eat at your desk - even if you only go away from your desk for a short time you will find you eat less if you are eating consciously.
10. Do have a 'kitchen cut off' time. Choose a reasonable time after which you choose not to eat. Be reasonable about it and make sure if you do eat after this time it is because you are genuinely hungry. Don't eat because it is late and you are tired and you think eating will give you more energy. Or because you have the munchies.

11. If it feels like you are dieting – stop – re read the rules and start again
12. Start creating your own handy hints as you go. Write them down in the space below – anything you think will help you.

The Hunger Scale Bit

Did you even know there is a recognised hunger scale?

Here it is – Most people eat when they are between a 3 and 5 on the hunger scale.

At **0**, you are empty. You might be feeling nauseous, dizzy, or light-headed

At **1**, you are ravenous. All you can think about is how hungry you are. Because you're so hungry, once you do eat, it's likely that you will over-eat to compensate.

At **2**, you are over-hungry. You've been thinking about food for a while now

At **3**, you are having hunger pangs. It's time to eat. Your body is giving you the natural signals that it needs food.

At **4**, your hunger is just starting to make itself known

At **5**, you are neutral. A little peckish maybe

At **6**, you are just satisfied. You aren't hungry anymore, but could manage a little more if it's tasty enough

At **7**, you are completely satisfied. You are no longer hungry.

At **8**, you are full. You have eaten a bit more than you need and fell a little bloated.

At **9**, you are overfull. You are uncomfortable

At **10**, you are stuffed and bloated. You feel awful. You are feel sick and might want to lie down until you feel better.

The Science Bit

If there was something in your body whose chief job was to make you feel hungry and something else that decreased your appetite I can guess which one you would want more of.

Often referred to as the hunger hormones, Ghrelin and Leptin are the hormones that fit this bill. There are complex interactions between them so I have tried to sum up a few of the most salient points. The other hormone that is currently attracting a lot of attention is cholecystoknin.

Ghrelin increases your appetite.

Ghrelin is released to signal hunger to the brain.

Ghrelin levels go up when your body requires nutrition. The problem here is that if you are not eating the right nutrient you body is asking for then the ghrelin levels do not drop.

If you imagine that your body needs protein and vitamins in addition to energy and you give it just sugar and fat. The urge for nutrients may be temporarily suppressed but does not go away so you find you are hungry again very shortly after you have snacked.

Ghrelin controls how quickly hunger comes back after we eat. Normally, ghrelin levels go up dramatically before you eat letting you know that you need energy and other nutrients. They go down again when you have eaten.

Leptin decreases your appetite.

Leptin tells your brain that the body has enough energy stores such as body fat. It helps with the maintenance of energy expenditure and metabolism.

Unfortunately the fatter you are, the more likely it is that your brain has learned to ignore these signals even though you have ample stores of fat.

Leptin levels are lower when if you are thin and higher if you are fatter. If you carry extra weight for a long time you can become resistant to the effects of Leptin.

On the down side Leptin can decrease (in a round about way) endorphins which leads to lower serotonin levels. Serotonin is also known as a happiness hormone because it contributes to feelings of well-being. It can have an inhibiting effect on your appetite .As we produce less Leptin when we are slimmer I guess we can look forward to feeling happier too.

In general, the fatter you are, the more Leptin is in your blood although the levels can change depending on when you last had something to eat and can also be affected by how much sleep you get.

We will investigate sleep again in a few pages time.

Cholecystokinin tells you when you have had enough

Cholecystokinin (CCK) is released in the duodenum and signals the brain to produce a sense of fullness. This happens particularly in response to high protein meals and meals with good quality fats.

Insulin turns the blood sugar into fat for storage.

Insulin. Insulin decides if blood sugar is used right immediately for energy or stored as fat. It is directly affected by our diets. The wrong combination of carbs fat and protein can lead to insulin resistance which can allow too much blood sugar or store too much as fat. Incorrect balance of some hormones, including insulin, can have a negative effect on your thyroid.

Adrenalin and cortisol – fight or flight reactors – can make you crave

Adrenalin and cortisol. Stress and anxiety can cause too much cortisol to be produced. This is part of your fight or flight reaction. It can cause cravings and binging as your body tries to build up energy for the impending crisis or restock after the sudden adrenalin usage.
Unfortunately the body cannot distinguish between physical danger – requiring more energy, and mental stress. So you stress eat.

Melatonin can influence Ghrelin and Leptin.

Melatonin can influence the production of ghrelin and leptin. Insufficient sleep can negatively affect your melatonin levels. (See the sleep bit)

Sleep

Sleep is more than just a convenient end to the day!

Without sleep brain function rapidly deteriorates. Sleep cycles are funkier and more complex than you think. First you have your non REM sleep and then your REM sleep (REM is rapid eye movement)

Most people experience about six to ten minutes of almost awake time followed by between half and one hour of deep sleep. Then you get around fifteen to twenty minutes of sleep where your brain waves increase.

The old adage about not eating before bed is all linked up with you needing ghrelin to get into this deep sleep brainwave zone and ghrelin levels drop for a few hours after eating. No ghrelin means no nice brainwavey sleep so your body will not do all those repairs and so forth that happen at night.

Once you get through the brainy sleep you get into the REM sleep. At this point your brain centre (it is called the suprachiasmatic nucleus but I like brain centre better) releases a chemical called hypocretin. One of its functions – the one we are most interested in – is to increase the release of leptin.

As explained above, this is the hormone that lets you know you have had enough and helps deal with excess. If you sleep only four hours instead of seven or eight hours your leptin is decreased by about forty to forty five percent. It also has a negative effect on your insulin resistance levels.

Not enough sleep means not enough leptin so if you wake up ravenous it is probable that you have not slept sufficiently.

Can we control the hunger hormones?

We can try!

Remember, persistence not perfection

We do not want to start over-thinking our food choices, that becomes a diet and we don't diet. Having said that, if there is some guidance it will help us out so a few tips on how to control hunger hormones can't hurt.

Research indicates that high protein foods and "good" carbohydrates (like whole grains) suppress ghrelin effectively

As mentioned before a good night's sleep will help suppress ghrelin levels. Plus if you are too tired your body tends to crave instant energy foods.

Evidence seems to point to good quality proteins and complex carbs being a good way to keep your body working for you rather than against you.

Fats, yes....fats.

Demonized since the eighties, the right fats do have a place in your eating habits so don't be scared of them. Cholecystokinin (CCK) is created in the duodenum when the cells there detect the presence of fat. It slows down the digestive process. CCK is also a neuropeptide so has direct access to the neurons in the brain to signal you are full. This is one reason fats are so important in the way you eat. Don't think no fats think good fats. (We have a whole chapter on this later).

After all – you are not on a diet and, to repeat myself; if it feels like you are, you are doing it wrong. You are on a bit of an adventure to discover how your body works so you can help it function nicely at the size and shape you want without too much effort.

Further on in this book there will be a list of friendly foods that help maintain hormone balance and help burn fats but here are a few that act as natural appetite suppressants.

Green Tea

Actually increases cholecystokinin (CCK) production – yup, the one that makes you feel full. That really is cheating. It does a whole bunch of other really good stuff but research suggests it can give you that full feeling, you usually only get with fats and protein, for up to two hours.

Apples

Apple pectin can help with keeping your blood sugar level and whilst making you feel as if you have eaten – the pectin prevents that blood sugar crash afterwards that can lead to cravings.

Bran

Yuk – but a couple of tablespoons of bran with a large glass of water can suppress your appetite for up to an hour with minimal calorific impact. It absorbs liquids in your stomach and makes you feel full. It does work but it is tricky to drink – worth it though.

Red wine vinegar/ cider vinegar

A couple of tablespoons in water is not going to taste very nice but is a small price to pay to help your blood sugar sustain its levels so you feel less hungry for an hour or two

Avocadoes

A tasty snack that does have a calorific impact but will keep you going as they stimulate CCK production.

Pine Nuts

Watch out for the calories but the pineolenic acid will stimulate CCK and quell those hunger pangs for a good half hour.

Almonds

Easy to snack on and also has those good fats to stimulate CCK for half an hour or so.

Water

Your body can be a bit daft when trying to tell the difference between hunger and thirst, fool it with a glass of water for a temporary stay of hunger pangs.

Taking advantage of any benefit you can get so you don't have to totally change you eating habits sounds like a good idea. These are a few friendly foods that assist in appetite suppression. Including some in moderation may assist you in controlling your appetite and therefore your weight. These are not miracle cures but any assistance is a bonus.

So bearing the above in mind you can persist in getting a grip on the hunger hormones and making them work with you and not against you. No diets just steady sustainable success.

The Personal Pep Talk Bit

You can do it – Go You

In reality I mean it. You actually can do it. You are the only one who can get rid yourself of excess weight and size.

Most poor eating habits start very young. Our natural programming is a bit animal in the fact that the very second we feel anything akin to hunger, we eat. Some of this is an instinctive urge to take advantage of a ready food source to insure us against times when food is scarce.

Some of it comes from childhood habits.

A baby cries and gets fed.

Food is comfort. Food makes us feel nice.

If you are my generation sweets were probably also a reward for good behaviour as a child.

Got to move on from that, I'm afraid.

Need to have a wee chat with the inner child and face the fact that behaviours formed from naught to six years old are not necessarily appropriate at *** years and ***stone.

Sit for a minute and really think about it. Think of all the things you have achieved. All the things you have learned.

How that marvellous piece of kit, your subconscious mind, can constantly direct you throughout your day.

So if you are that good, and everyone is, have a bit of a pep talk with it about listening to your body and only eating when you are actually hungry.

It would probably not do you too much harm to sit quietly each morning and having a bit of a self-talk about how you are going to get through the day easily and without over doing the eating. Even just reminding yourself to have one cookie instead of two or, if you are very brave, cut out both cookies!

This bit does sound crazy but the person you are most likely to listen to is you so maybe try a little self-pep talk. I took it a stage further and for positive reinforcement I recorded myself repeating the following sentences for about ten minutes and I regularly listen to it when I am on the train to work or even cooking or doing things around the house.

Eat when you are hungry, only when you are hungry
Eat slowly and mindfully
And when you have had enough, stop.

Ten minutes of that and I have switched off my brain to it completely but I really feel it has shoved itself somewhere into my subconscious.
I genuinely find myself putting down my knife and fork between mouthfuls which is something I would never have done historically.
Remember, you are not on a diet; you are just changing a few bits and bobs so you lose weight effortlessly, slowly and permanently.

Right now you need to have a talk with yourself. Think about it, since all you are doing is changing a few little bits about the way you eat there is no conceivable reason why you should not expect to be reducing your weight and size little by little, ounce by ounce, ounces become pounds; pounds become stone. Nothing drastic from day to day but an overall result over the next year or so. You can be sure of this if you follow the six rules and just become a bit more mindful of what, when and why your are eating.
It will happen, so ignore your inner critic and get on with it!

On the subject of your inner critic.....

To be really successful in anything you need to become aware of the internal 'chat' that goes on between your subconscious and conscious. Learn to recognise any negative thoughts and silence that inner critic.

By this I mean the whole negative chat you hear when you are about to scoff something when you are not hungry.

- ➤ What is the point I am never going to lose weight?
- ➤ I haven't lost any this week
- ➤ I've gained a few pounds so I might as well.
- ➤ I don't see why I should restrict myself
- ➤ I just want it
- ➤ I don't have any will power
- ➤ It's a shame to waste it
- ➤ It doesn't seem to make any difference.

Listen to your inner critic and then tell it to shut up.
Your inner critic does not have to rule your life.
Sometimes you need to be tough on yourself and just face the fact that you get to choose between having one extra slice of cake/glass of wine and being a few stone slimmer in several months in a way that will last for the rest of your life.
Treat your inner critic and all the negative talk and temptations like a pestering child tell it 'No' for its own sake. If you had an overweight child or pet you would feel responsible for their health – you owe at least as much to your own body.

You choose when and what you want to eat not some inner unconscious urge. Take control.

The 'What you should know about weight management' bit.

This will all sound very diet oriented but there are a few plain old facts you need if you are to understand how your weight will decrease without major restrictions.

To gain weight you take in more fuel than you use in energy.

I hate referring to calories but that is the standard to measure the body's fuel/energy system so I am afraid I will have to use it.

Below is a table that indicates the amount of calories per day to maintain a specific weight in the average reasonably inactive style.

From this you can get an idea of the deficit between what you need to sustain your current size. If you don't want to sustain your current size – this at least puts thing into proportion but I still don't want you to get hung up on these figures but you need a basic idea of how your body uses and stores energy.

This figure decreases over the age of 60 but the below is a guide.

If your intake is less than your body need to function you will lose weight.

The table below is approximate.

Weight	Men	Women
9 stone	1970	1700
10 stone	2070	1760
11 stone	2160	1830
12 stone	2260	1900
13 stone	2360	1960
14 stone	2450	2030
15 stone	2540	2100
16 stone	2640	2160
17 stone	2730	2260
18 stone	2830	2330
19 stone	2930	2360
20 stone	3020	2460

21 stone	3110	2500
22 stone	3200	2560
23 stone	3300	2630
24 stone	3400	2700
25 stone	3500	2760

One pound in weight reduction takes a deficit of three thousand five hundred calories. To get rid of one pound in seven days you need to intake five hundred calories per day, on average, less than you are using.

This may seem a lot but if you relate this to long term non goal specific weight reduction and think more of getting rid of between half a pound and a pound a week .

If you think about shedding half a pound a week that is still twenty six pounds in a year.

To get rid of only half a pound a week would be a reduction of two hundred and fifty calories a day. You could cut one small thing out – that semi skimmed latte and a cookie for instance (or in my case pint of cider) - and already be on track without really thinking about it.

Here are 20 foods with the low calorific values per 100 grams

Celery 26	Blueberries 53
Tomatoes 17	Asparagus 20
Cucumber 16	Lemons 29
Cauliflower 25	Mushrooms 40
Apples 52	Broccoli 34
Grapefruit 42	Onions 40
Cabbage 25	Spinach 20
Watermelon 30	Watercress 11
Cherries 51	Oranges 47

Compare that with
Butter 735
Sugar 397

Calorific value of basic nutrition.

Fat = 9 calories per gram
Protein = 4 calories per gram
Carbs = 4 calories per gram

So if you know fat, protein and carbs in a food you can work out how many calories that food contains.

Up your outlay of energy by just a little and reduce your intake by just a little and the weight and size will reduce without too much trouble. Stop expecting the diet industry to work miracles and take charge.

The exercise bit

Do some.

Walk up the stairs instead of using the lift.

If your knees are dodgy find somewhere safe to cycle – I bought a second hand exercise bike for fifteen pounds in a charity shop.

Walk up from the station instead of getting the bus

Get off the bus a stop early and walk.

Go for a walk at lunchtime.

Go swimming – my local pool used to have an adults only evening a couple of times a week – smilingly referred to as the Happy Hippos............

Walk around the block at least once a day.

It's a start.

Get into the habit of doing something a little more than you currently do every day.

Go join a gym if you like that sort of thing.

Buy a swing ball for the back garden.

Join a salsa class.

Just do something that gets you moving a bit – who knows, you might enjoy it.

To give you a brief idea I have to use the calorie word again

Exercise	How long it takes to burn 250 calories
Walking	60 minutes
Cycling	30 minutes
Yoga	85 minutes
Running	40 minutes
Gardening	60 minutes
Netball	50 minutes
Housework – active	80 minutes
Cross trainer	40 minutes
Skipping	40 minutes

I'm afraid it's that whole choice thing again – add a little movement or be bigger than you would like to. We are not looking for a quick fix so you don't have to go crazy but a little extra exercise will lead to a little less you.

If you don't want to diet – you need to get a bit of movement going.

The NLP/Mindfulness bit.

Neuro Linguistic Programming, or NLP as it is more commonly referred to as, is the study of the way the human brain reacts to reality experience and verbal expression. Often used in businesses in relation to increasing ones influencing skill it originated as a method of achieving personal excellence. There are some basic assumptions of NLP can help us understand our cravings and our behaviours.

1. **We react to experience rather than reality** – for example our experience tells us a certain food is associated with reward and comfort– we eat this food when we need to reward ourselves whether we are hungry or not. We may even crave this food and convince ourselves we are hungry to justify eating it when in reality we just want to feel nice and rewarded.

2. **The resources an individual needs to effect change are already within them.** – You are in control and you are totally capable of persisting in this determination to follow the rules and get to your ideal size and shape.

3. **If you always do what you have always done you will always get what you have always got.** – You got fat – so it's time to change something in the way you have been doing things. You don't have to diet but something has to change and only you can decide what.

4. **The positive worth of an individual is constant it is the external behaviour that can be questionable.** – You are a terrific person. You worth does not equate to your size and shape. You have allowed yourself to get out of shape but that does not make you bad. You have decided now to address this and get a responsible relationship with food.

5. **There is a positive intention motivating every behaviour.** – Something in your relationship with food makes, or has made, you feel good. So let's see if there is a better way to get those good feelings.

6. **Feedback vs. failure- All results and behaviours are achievements**. Every poor food choice is a

reminder to get back on track. Every slip up is a reason to get back to taking care of yourself. Don't be too hard on yourself – be a friend and a coach and laugh at you mistakes whilst learning from them. Persistence not perfection.

Mindfulness is a concept that encourages practitioners to become centred in the moment and be fully aware of what they are doing and how their minds and bodies are responding to both internal and external influences. By being aware of what you are doing and why you can bring about changes in a permanent and positive way. Be aware of why you are eating – actually hungry or filling some other need. Eating mindfully, knowing why you are eating, and enjoying the moment and flavours and textures. Put your attention on what you are doing so you know when to stop.

Both of these methods / concepts are relevant in relation to why we eat when we are not actually hungry. If you want to get a grip on your motivation for eating these ideas will help immensely.
Emotional eating is triggered by our reaction to external influences and remembered experience using food as a reward or comfort or even to fill and emotional emptiness. Admittedly some food will release endorphins that actually make you feel better but none of these feelings will equal the good feelings you will have as you slowly and permanently melt away the excess pounds.

Thinking back to the pep talk – the best pep talk you can give can only come from you. You are the only person who really understands why you eat erratically or emotionally when you can be fully aware that you are not actually hungry.
Next time you reach for the biscuits, chocolate or in my case cheese ask yourself what you are feeling. Sit down put the food in front of you and try to understand why that food is the one you feel you need even though you are not hungry. How does it make you feel? Why do you need to feel that way? Is there an

alternative way of getting the same feeling? If you can learn to question yourself in relation to your food choices you can start to understand them. Once you understand them you can take control.

When I get a cheese craving I imagine the cheese covered in baked beans, my worst ever food, if I still fancy it then I know I am truly hungry. If I have gone off the idea I then know I was having and emotional craving.

Persistence not perfection.

I know I say it a lot but you could do worse than repeat it to yourself every day. It seems to be in the spring when layers get less and you might want to get a bit of skin out that the urge to diet grabs you – RESIST!

No dieting, remember? Diets fail, restrictions make you feel rotten, and goals set you up to feel bad. You can do it, in your own time, in your own way. If you must think 'lose weight for spring' think next spring. Remember half a pound a week and you will be two stone lighter this time next year so stop stressing about food, eat when you are hungry, eat slowly, stop when you have had enough, make a few simple changes and stop beating yourself up for being overweight.

Sustainable weight loss not sudden weight loss.

Try this.
1. Picture yourself this time next year – a couple of stone lighter, slimmer and fitter. Imagine the things you will be able to do – not might, will- imagine yourself at your ideal weight and size – close your eyes and really picture it – how good does that feel?
2. Seriously think about a realistic size and shape – not how you were when you were in your teens – that's probably unrealistic – think about just one size down. Don't think tiny: think less than I am now is an achievement. No goals, remember. Just an idea of being trimmer. Not super model just smaller and fitter than now.

3. Decide who you will tell. Some friends may love you as you are and be threatened by your decision to change. This sounds crazy but humans are strange that way and within relationships many people find change threatening. You will know who will truly support you but make it clear to them that telling you 'you are fine as you are' is not the sort of support you need.
4. Find a way to reward yourself that does not involve food. Manicure, hair appointment, movies – something to make you feel rewarded. Couple of hours of Xbox/ play station.

The 'What on earth is Thermogenic food?' bit

Thermogenic foods are your friends!
These are foods that take maximum energy for your body to digest. Some can take almost as many calories as they contain. The word thermogenic comes from the fact they raise your body temp. They also help to increase your metabolism and as they take longer to digest. The energy is released over a longer period of time so you feel less hungry.
Also, to get technical, a portion of dietary calories in excess of those required for immediate energy requirements are converted to heat rather than stored as fat.
In theory, if you eat a thermogenic food, your core temperature will increase and also cause your metabolism to speed up. A faster metabolism translates into more calories being burned. So you quite literally burn it off!
It is not a miracle weight loss secret or anything but for the purpose of long term sustainable weight control it certainly does not hurt.

Here are a few thermogenic foods. On the left are the herbs and spices on the right are the more substantial foods. Quite a few of these will also appear in the chapter addressing super foods. There is a crossover between the super foods groups and the thermogenic ones.
Remember, they are not miracle workers but any advantage you can get is a bonus.

Chilli peppers	Grapefruit
Black pepper	Celery
Turmeric	Coconut oil
Cinnamon	Broccoli
Cardamom	Cauliflower
Basil	Brussels sprouts
Garlic	Kale
Ginger	Cabbage
Green Tea	Lean protein (fish,

	chicken/turkey breast)
Cider Vinegar	Asparagus
Ice water	Berries

From the above it should be quite easy to put together a 'fat burning' menu or at least try to do a few swapsies for things you currently eat or drink.

If you don't want to diet – you take any advantage you can get!

The 'What about fat?' bit

Not all fats are created equal

Demonised for many years, whilst we have been steered towards a low fat eating regime that is now being criticised for being ineffective, fats fall into four main groups.

- monounsaturated fats
- polyunsaturated fats
- saturated fats
- trans fats

Monounsaturated fats and polyunsaturated fats are **good** for you as they assist in lowering cholesterol and reducing you risk of heart disease.

Trans fats and saturated fats are **bad** and will raise your cholesterol and increase your risk of heart disease

The difference between good and bad fats

Trans fats and saturated fats are responsible for the bad rap fats have got over the years and are guilty of adding to weight gain, clogged arteries, and so forth.

Monounsaturated fats, polyunsaturated fats, and omega-3s are not only **not** guilty of the above but are actually healthy and help you manage your moods, keep your brain healthy, fight fatigue, and even control your weight.

Your body needs fats; you just need to just learn the good from the bad.

Good fats vs. bad fats.

To break it down to its simplest components – here is another list

Good Fats	
Monounsaturated fats	**Polyunsaturated fats**
Olive oil	Soybean oil
Sunflower oil	Linseed / Flaxseed oil
Sesame oil	Corn oil
Peanut oil	Soy milk
Almond oil	Tofu
Almonds	Almond milk
Peanut butter	Fish oils and oily fish
Most nuts and associated oils	Walnuts
Avocados	Safflower oil
Olives	Seeds – sesame, sunflower, pumpkin
Bad Fats	
Saturated Fat	**Trans Fats**
Fat on meat – lamb, beef, pork	Cakes, biscuits, pastries, pizzas, pies
Chicken skin	Chips, crisps, popcorn, savoury snacks
Lard	Sweets and chocolate
Cheese	Anything fried
Milk	Ice cream, custards and sauces
Cream	Margarine and spreads
Butter	Processed desserts
Palm oil	Take-aways (most of them)
Coconut oil	Anything you really really like

Bad fats

Saturated vs. Trans

Excessive consumption of saturated fat can raise blood cholesterol levels and increases the risk of heart disease and stroke. It would be a good idea to cut down where possible and exchange the saturated for something in the good fat selection. A moderate amount is not fantastic if you want to maintain your figure either but for all over health change a few of them to help your body function at its best.

No amount of trans fats is healthy. Trans fats contribute to major health problems, from heart disease to cancer. They are fat molecules treated with hydrogen to make them last longer. This does not improve your food quality or enjoyment but it does extend their sell by date – good for the retailer, not so good for your body. The word 'hydrogenated' or 'partially hydrogenated' means trans fats. Become a trans-fat avoidance specialist to increase your general health, help your body perform better and get to that ideal you. Be nice to your body and you will feel the excess weight melt away.

Reduce your intake of bad fats – cut out trans fats where possible and find more pleasure in eating and being both healthier and trimmer. (Slowly, of course – we don't want to diet, now)

Omega-3 fatty acids

I will mention omega 3 again in the nutrition bit but take note of this extremely healthy fat it can do all the below and more (allegedly)

- ✓ Prevent and reduce the symptoms of depression
- ✓ Protect against memory loss and dementia
- ✓ Reduce the risk of heart disease, stroke, and cancer
- ✓ Ease symptoms of arthritis, joint pain, and inflammatory skin conditions

Get some in if you know what's good for you

The 'What about Sugar' Bit

Added sugar contains no nutritional value and is bad for your teeth. It is empty calories and added sugars tend to be high in fructose which can cause issues for your liver.

Sugar and your liver

When you intake sugar it is broken down in your digestive tract into two main constituents glucose and fructose. Glucose is essential within the body and you would produce it if you do not have enough but fructose is a substance for which the body has little use. Your liver will turn fructose into fat and most of it gets stored it in your fat cells. Some of it does not leave your liver and can cause non-alcoholic fatty liver disease.

Sugar and your insulin levels

Insulin facilitates the burning of glucose as energy instead of burning fat as energy. Insulin allows glucose to be absorbed by your cells to be burned. Too much glucose in the blood is very bad. When you have too much glucose your cells can become resistant to insulin. This is linked to obesity, heart disease, metabolic syndrome and type two diabetes.

Sugar and diabetes

If your cells become resistant to insulin your body (your pancreas) makes more of it as your body thinks you have a deficiency but as you become more and more resistant to insulin your blood sugar levels rise to a toxic level. This is when you may well be diagnosed with type two diabetes.

Sugar (fructose) and appetite

Research suggests that fructose does not have the same effect on your appetite as glucose. You will not feel satisfied as your ghrelin level will be insufficiently lowered. (see the hunger hormones bit)

Sugar and you brain.

Sugar consumption can release high levels of dopamine in the brain, giving you a 'sugar high'. This high, like any, can be very addictive. The feel good factor of sugar laced foods can lead to cravings that can be hard to resist. You can kick this 'habit' only by stopping completely. It is possible to virtually eliminate most sugar from your eating habits.

Sugar and heart disease.

Sugar is becoming the No1 enemy in the fight against heart disease. High amounts of fructose can raise blood glucose levels and cholesterol.
Sugar and obesity

After years of being told that a low fat diet will cure obesity it is now widely agreed that sugar not fat consumption is the leading cause of the obesity epidemic. What makes it so ironic is that in so many low fat foods the fat has been replaced with sugar to assist in enhancing the flavour.

Artificial sweeteners and other sugar substitutes.

So if you are trying to get rid of sugar – what can you do to make life a bit sweeter?

Here are some options along with a mixture of research and opinions that (allegedly) relate to them.

Artificial sweeteners

Manufactured and synthesised from various components, some natural - some not so, these are usually the intensely sweet substitutes you get in fizzy drinks when the words sugar free are used. They usually have an extremely low calorific value and turn up in processed food and drinks. They are assumed to be beneficial to weight management due to their low or negligible calorie content. They also have negligible effect on blood sugar and so are considered suitable for diabetics. Some of them have been speculatively linked to a variety of diseases but scientific proof is sketchy and they are considered generally safe. Public opinion varies greatly so you need to make up your own mind if generally safe is good enough. Artificial sweeteners include acesulfame, saccharin, aspartame, neotame and sucralose.

Natural sweeteners

I am using natural to include sweeteners that are not chemical based.

Stevia is quite new to the market and is refined from a naturally grown plant but contains zero calories in its refined form it is 200 to 300 times sweeter than sugar but has zero effect on your blood sugar. Stevia is currently the market favourite. (And mine!)

Agave nectar is also plant based, coming from the same plant that gives us tequila, contains a probiotic that helps the good bacteria in your stomach. It is a syrup from the root of the plant but whilst has more calories than sugar it is much sweeter so you need considerably less.

Honey has about 80 fewer calories than sugar per 100 grams but its major benefit comes from the fact that whilst sugar contains very little else, honey contains a little dietary fibre, vitamins C, B3, B5, B12 , choline and betaine – if only in trace amounts. It also has calcium, iron, selenium, zinc, manganese, magnesium, phosphorus, potassium and sodium so comparatively speaking it is nutritionally far more valuable than sugar. Calorifically it is not such a winner but from a nutritional perspective you should consider it a valid substitute.

Coconut sugar comes from evaporating the water out of sap from the coconut plant – this is not the same as palm sugar. It does retain some of the nutrients of the coconut and contains iron, calcium, some antioxidants and potassium. It also contains a bit much fructose so although it is a viable replacement for processed white sugar it is still not as good as stevia or cutting out sugar altogether. It has the same calorific value as standard sugar.

Blackstrap molasses contains 100 calories per 100 grams less than sugar and contains vitamin B's and also calcium, iron, magnesium, phosphorus, potassium, sodium, zinc, copper, manganese, selenium in trace amounts but has a more acidic flavour than standard sugar. It is slightly better from a calorific perspective and has a much better nutritional value.

Yacon Syrup is extracted from the Yacon which is indigenous to Brazil, Bolivia, and Peru. Yacon is considered the best sweetener because it contains more than 50 percent FOS (Fructooligosacharides), which does not in any way increase blood glucose levels. So it is good for both dieting and diabetics. It has a flavour similar to molasses or caramel but negligible calorific value.

Sugar alcohols

Sugar alcohols, sometimes called polyols, occur naturally in certain fruits and vegetables and are a type of carbohydrate, They are generally about the same or less sweet than sugar itself but they are considerably lower in calories. They are beneficial due to the lower calorie content and they have minimum impact on blood sugar and can be found in many diabetic foods. They tend to be added to processed food and drink to replace sugar but do beware as excess consumption can have a laxative effect. If you see this warning on something, it probably contains polyols. They come in the guise of hydrogenated starch, isomalt, lactitol, maltitol, sorbitol, xylitol but are often just referred to as polyols.

The eating clean food bit

Many processed foods can inhibit weight reduction. Even those promoted as low fat along with the insinuation that they are healthy will contain something to replace the fat content. On many occasions this will be sugar. The food loses taste when the fat content is reduced and the sugar will enhance the flavour.

Many foods that initially look healthy have lost much of their positive nutritional value due to over processing.
If you can reheat it in a microwave to eat it, you will probably have destroyed much of the nutritional value just in the double cooking process. When a food is sold from the chiller in a supermarket – check the storage instructions. If it is labelled 'best served chilled' or 'refrigerate after opening' rather than instructing you to store it in the fridge immediately then it is probably worth checking the label to see what is preserving it so well.

I get that you probably like a few convenience foods but ultimately if you want to easily and slowly and permanently manage your weight you need to be aware of what you are eating.
Even flavourings can be deceiving. Some natural vanilla flavourings (not all, I might add) are derived from the secretions from the anal glands of a species of beaver. E120 is ground up beetles. Whilst these two examples will not affect your weight – you might find looking into what you are eating brings some surprising facts. When the word 'natural' is used be on guard – whilst beaver butt juice (castoreum) is natural, I'm not convinced you want it on the menu.
The fresher the better – really want to maintain that ideal weight and size? Learn to cook. Once you know what you are eating and start caring about what you put in your body you will find it much easier to make choices.

In addition you will find that you can produce meals that contain exactly what you want them too and taste really good. It can also work out cheaper once you know what you are doing. Clean food – if you feel the urge to go crazy organic on it – do it! It's not my bag I just try to keep eating clean food where possible.

Keep it cleaner and you will end up leaner

Here are some of the more common additives and where they come from. All are allegedly harmless but I'm not sure how many of them you really want to eat.

Firstly they are grouped by what they do. The additives that you are most likely to come across on food labels are:

Antioxidants
Colours
Emulsifiers
Stabilisers, gelling agents and thickeners
Flavour enhancers
Preservatives
Of the above only the flavour enhancers are really there to enhance your eating experience. The rest are basically to keep food on the shelves for longer. Making it last increases its saleability. This is fine and understandable from a marketing and profit perspective but it is not being done for your benefit.

Here are a few derived from bits of animals and a few other unsavoury items.

E-number	Name	Origin
E120	Carmine, Cochineal	Colour isolated from the insects *Coccus cacti* Cochineal is the result of crushing scales of the insect into a red powder.
E153	Carbon Black	Likely to be derived from various parts of animals.
E161	Canthaxanthin	Although Canthaxanthin is usually derived from plant material, it can sometimes be made from fish and invertebrates with hard shells.
E252	Potassium Nitrate	Usually of natural origins but potassium nitrate can be artificially manufactured from waste animal matter.
E322	Lecithine	Soy beans and for some purposes from chicken eggs.
E441	Gelatin	From animal bones. Since the BSE crisis mainly from pork, but other animal bones are used. Halal gelatin is available in specialised shops.
E474	Sugarglycerides	Combination of sugar and fatty acids.
E485	Gelatine	From animal bones. Since the BSE crisis mainly from pork, but other animal bones are used.
E542	Edible bone phosphate	From animal bones. Since the BSE crisis mainly from pork, but other animal bones are used.
E626-29	Guanylic acid and guanylatens	Mainly from yeast, also from sardines and meat.
E630-35	Inosinic acid and inosinates	Mainly from meat and fish, also made with bacteria.

E631	Disodium inosinate -	Flavour enhancer Almost always made from animals and fish
E636, E637	Maltol and Isomaltol	From malt (barley), sometimes also from heating milk sugar.
E640	Glycin	Mainly from gelatine (see 441 above), also synthetically.
E901	Bees wax	Made by bees, but does not contain insects.
E904	Shellac	Natural polymer derived from certain species of lice from India. Insects get trapped in the resin.
E913	Lanolin	A wax from sheep. It is excreted by the skin of the sheep and extracted from the wool.
E920-21	Cystein en cystin	Derived from proteins, including animal protein and hair.
E966	Lactitol	Made from milk sugar
E1000	Cholic acid	From beef (bile)
E1105	Lysozym	From chicken eggs

So, whilst much of the above is harmless but ....YUK

The Nutrition bit

All this talk of what is bad for you but no one really explains what is good for you and why. We all know the basics with protein and carbs but what about all the bits in between. Here is a bit of a breakdown of some of the other nutrients essential for your health. It gives an idea of what we are looking for in our eating plans. I'm tired of people referring to super foods etc whilst up until researching this book I did not really understand why a food was super and what it actually does.

Antioxidants

Lots of foods are rich in antioxidants – which is great. But why? Antioxidants protect your cells from the damaging effects of these things called free radicals. Free radicals are everywhere, in the air, our bodies, and the materials around us. They cause the deterioration of plastics, the fading of paint, the degradation of works of art, aging related illnesses, and can contribute to heart attacks, stroke and cancers. (freeradical.org.au) Antioxidants are generally believed to be the good guys in the fight against many diseases and are under research in relation to Alzheimer's, cystic fibrosis and memory loss.
Beta-carotene, lycopene, lutein, selenium, and vitamins A, C, and E all fall into the antioxidant category.

Omega 3

I was always hearing about it but I only had a vague idea what it did until I started research. It has already had a mention in this book but it is worth a second one. It is simply an essential fatty acid found in fish oil, eggs and flaxseed amongst others. Your body cannot make omega-3 but as it can lower blood pressure, reduce the risk of cardiovascular disease, stroke and cancer help lower triglyceride levels, help treat the inflammatory symptoms of rheumatoid arthritis and other inflammatory diseases including inflammatory skin conditions it is certainly worth including in your eating plan. It can also improve brain function and assist with symptoms of depression, protect against memory loss and dementia.

Vitamins

Vitamin A

As well as the antioxidant benefits, vitamin A maintains healthy eyes, good vision, immune system, reproductive system and strong bones and teeth. It supports normal cell growth.

Vitamin B

The seven types of B vitamins play an essential role in breaking down food into a usable energy form. They work together targeting proteins fats and carbs to maintain a healthy balance within your body although each has a speciality, as it were.

B1 and B2 (thiamin and riboflavin) assist with energy production but have a specific effect on the function of the heart, muscles and nerves.

B3 (niacin) works to maintain healthy skin, nervous system and digestion.

B5 (pantothenic acid) is essential in normal growth and cell development.

B6 (pyridoxine) builds blood cells, supports the immune system, the nervous system and assists in the breakdown of proteins.

B7 (*biotin)* assists with breaking down protein and carbohydrates and supports healthy hormone production

B9 (*folic acid* or *folate)* is essential in blood cell production and as it also makes and maintains DNA it is essential in pregnancy.

B12 (cobalamin) builds blood cells, supports the immune system, the nervous system and assists in the breakdown of carbohydrates. It is also essential for cell development and normal growth

Vitamin C

Another antioxidant but this one not only supports the immune system and can help fight infections. It also looks after bones and teeth and assists in creating the collagen that keeps your skin healthy and repairs and heals wounds.

Vitamin D

Your body needs vitamin D to absorb calcium and phosphorus. It also boosts the immune system has a beneficial anti-inflammatory effect , may reduce risk of cancer and due to its interaction with calcium and phosphorus maintains bone integrity and even can assist in the prevention of bone loss due to osteoporosis.

Vitamin E

Antioxidant packed vitamin E helps the body use some of the other vitamins more efficiently, supports red blood cell formation and boosts the immune system.

Vitamin K

Vitamin K is essential for your blood to clot properly. It assists in building the right sort of proteins and also helps maintain bone integrity.

Minerals

Calcium

Calcium is a main component of building and maintaining strong healthy bones and teeth. It is well known for these qualities but is also vital in protecting the brain, heart and lungs. It assists in the protection of muscles and nerves and is essential for blood clotting.

Choline

Only recently recognised as an essential mineral this is being researched in relation to beneficial effects on building DNA, exchanging signals in the brain, and detoxification in your liver.

Chromium

Another little known mineral that we do not need a lot of but is essential to enable our bodies make use of fats and carbohydrates. Chromium is good for cholesterol management and assists in the metabolism of insulin.

Copper

Only required in very small amount and mostly stored in your liver this trace mineral is found in every tissue of your body and is vital to stay healthy. It assists in the creation of red blood cells and melanin, looks after your skin by assisting in the production of collagen and helps keep your immune system healthy.

Iodine

Another trace mineral, this one is stored in the thyroid gland and enables your body to turn food into energy.

Iron

It's everywhere! Found in the liver, spleen, red blood cells, bone marrow and muscles it helps to build proteins in your blood. This in turn enables oxygen to be moved around your body keeping you alive and healthy and energised. You could not function without it

Magnesium

We need a lot of this multifunctional mineral. It helps iron with the production of the oxygen transporting proteins and works with calcium to support nerves and muscles. It is found in most tissues and many of your organs. It is very active in assisting heart function.

Manganese

A trace mineral that impacts bone formation, skin health, can impact blood sugar and protects against free radicals and still most people have never heard of it!

Molybdenum

This trace element enables our bodies to utilise nitrogen from the air and also plays a part in helping iron with the oxygen distribution to your cells. It helps maintain cell membranes too and also assists in protecting your teeth.

Potassium

This is needed for many functions as it assists in the control of fluid balance and regulates the kidney efficiency and moves fluids around the cells in your body. Your body also needs it for muscle contractions and nerve responses. It is essential for both brain and heart maintenance and repair functions and maintaining overall good health.

Phosphorus

Strangely enough phosphorus is one of the minerals we need a lot of just to run the body on a day to day basis. Phosphorus works with calcium to build bones and teeth but is also a main component of our direct genetic material. It assists in the breakdown of carbohydrate, fat and protein but also assists the kidneys in filtering and removing waste from the body. It supports the build and repair of tissues and cells and not only aids the storing of energy but also helps to keep you heart in good condition.

Selenium

Whilst we need very little selenium, it is essential in the functioning of the immune system and thyroid gland. It has an antioxidant effect by building and maintaining proteins that assist in the protection of individual cells.

Zinc

You need a substantial amount of this nutrient to stay healthy. Not only does it boost your immune but also assists in the creation of proteins that are the DNA building blocks of your genetic makeup. It assists your bodies healing process and also in the maintenance of both your sense of smell and taste.

The Super foods Bit

Strictly speaking there is no such thing as a superfood. This must be true because EU legislation no longer allows any food package to use superfood on its label so below are a list foods that pack a nutritional punch some of which were formerly known as 'super'.

Almonds

Nuts are a food rich in healthy fats.
Almonds in particular can help you shed pounds. A daily helping of the nuts to replace a processed snack will have an immediate effect on your health and your waistline. High in monounsaturated fats associated with reduced risk of heart disease they also have cholesterol lowering qualities. They contain vitamins E and B2, B3, manganese, copper, phosphorus, magnesium and molybdenum. Eating almonds can quite possibly reduce your risk of gaining weight too.

Apples

Apples are full of antioxidants. They are also full of vitamin C for healthy skin and gums. They also contain a form of soluble fibre called pectin that can help to lower blood cholesterol levels and keep the digestive system healthy.

Apricots

Apricots are full of beta-carotene and fibre. Nutrients in apricots can help protect the heart and eyes. Apricots are also a good source of vitamins A and C, copper and potassium.

Asparagus

Particularly effective in assisting in the removal of waste products, asparagus contains Vitamins K, B1,B2,C,B3,A and B6 it also has traces of B9, copper, selenium, manganese, phosphorus, potassium, choline, zinc, iron, protein, B5, magnesium and calcium.

Basically it is brilliant.

Some varieties contain phytonutrient called saponins. Saponins have been shown to have anti-inflammatory and anti-cancer properties, and their intake has also been associated with improved blood pressure, improved blood sugar regulation, and better control of blood fat levels.

They also contain inulin. Inulin encourages certain types of bacteria in the intestine that lower risk of allergy and lower risk of colon cancer.

Avocados

Do not be scared of fats, just choose the right ones. Oleic acid can stimulate cholecystokinin (CCK) production in your body to actually quiet hunger. Oleic acid can increase our absorption of fat-soluble nutrients like carotenoids. It can also help lower our risk of heart disease. They have anti-inflammatory properties like no other food and can assist in the prevention of arthritis. They contain vitamins K, B5, B6 B9, E, C, potassium, and copper. Alpha-carotene, beta-carotene, beta-cryptoxanthin, chrysanthemaxanthin, lutein, neochrome, neoxanthin, violaxanthin, zeaxanthin.

Bananas

Bananas are slightly higher in energy and therefore calories than some other fruits but the carbohydrate level restores energy and the high nutritional density ensures them a place on a super foods list. They are beneficial in the lowering of blood pressure due to the high potassium level and a satisfying snack in moderation. Bananas contain Vitamins B6, B7 and C, manganese, potassium, and copper in addition to fibre.

Beetroot

Beetroot is a unique source of phytonutrients called betalains. They provide antioxidant, anti-inflammatory, and detoxification support. They also contribute to eye health and have a beneficial effect on the nervous system. They are almost incredibly rich in antioxidants. They contain manganese, potassium, copper, magnesium, phosphorus, vitamins C and B6, B9 and iron.

Bell Peppers (sweet peppers)

Bell peppers area source of over 30 different members of the carotenoid nutrient family. They provide antioxidant and anti-inflammatory health benefits. There is ongoing research into their potential anti-cancer benefits.
They contain Vitamins C, A, B6, E, B2, K, B1, B6, B9, molybdenum, potassium, manganese and magnesium

Black Pepper

Black pepper can assist in your digestive processes and reduce the incidence of heartburn. It assists in detoxification by promoting sweating and being a diuretic (making you pee). The outside of a peppercorn help breakdown your fat cells. It contains vitamin K, chromium, iron and manganese.

Black beans

Black beans contain 15 grams of protein per one hundred grams and contain no saturated fat. As a fill source of fibre. Black beans keep the intestine and colon healthy and can lower the risk of this form of cancer. They contain Iron, folate, magnesium, protein, vitamin B1, manganese, copper and fibre.

Blueberries

High fibre, low calorie and have anti-aging properties. They have one of the highest antioxidant capacities among all fruits, vegetables, spices and seasonings. Particularly efficient in assisting with maintenance of brain health consumption, over time, can assist with memory issues. They contain vitamins K and C, manganese, copper and fibre.

Brazil nuts

Brazil nuts are one of the few good sources of selenium that may help protect against cancer, depression and Alzheimer's disease.

Broccoli

Cooked or raw, broccoli is well known for its anti-cancer and cholesterol lowering benefits. It has a very strong detoxification effect with phytonutrients that assist eliminating toxins and help your system at a genetic level. Generally considered one of the most nutrient rich vegetables broccoli contains Vitamins K,C,B6,E,B2,A,B1,B3, selenium, B9, iron, zinc, calcium, chromium, B5, manganese, choline, potassium, magnesium and copper

Brown rice

Whole grains generally, including brown rice, have been investigated in relation to protection from colon cancer, high cholesterol and even type 2 diabetes. It is packed full of antioxidants and is rich in fibre. It contains vitamin B3, copper, manganese, selenium, magnesium, fibre and phosphorus.

Brussels sprouts

Love them or hate them you can't ignore the health benefits of these amazing little vegetables. They have cholesterol lowering properties and have a beneficial effect on white blood cells. Along with anti-carcinogenic properties they contain vitamins K, C, B1, B2 ,B3, B6 and A and calcium, magnesium, protein, B9, manganese, fibre, choline, copper, omega 3 fats, iron, potassium, phosphorus, B5 and zinc.

Cauliflower

Cauliflower has been studied for its cancer-preventing potential and antioxidant properties. Additionally it is linked to anti-inflammatory properties, may offer cardiovascular support and has high fibre so supports your digestive tract health. Cauliflower has dense nutritional value containing vitamins C, K, B6, B2, B1, B3, B9, and B5, choline, omega 3 fats, manganese, B7, potassium, protein and magnesium.

Cherries

Cherries are one of those nutritional super foods that you should eat whenever available. Containing good levels of melatonin they have been linked with reducing cancer and heart disease and as melatonin is a natural sleep aid can assist with this as well. They contain a natural chemical (anthocyanins) which can help your skin stay looking good. They have been linked to reduction of pain from both arthritis and gout due to their anti_-inflammatory properties. High in water and low in fat they can also assist you to burn fat more effectively. They contain B9, B3, B5, B6, B2, B1, vitamins C, E, A, K, potassium, sodium, calcium, copper, iron, magnesium, manganese, phosphorus and zinc.

Chia seeds

High in antioxidants and fibre, with the added slimming benefit of most of the carb content being fibre, chia seeds are a high quality protein but also due to the fibre content these helpful seeds absorb much of the liquid in your digestive system and bulk out to make you feel full. They are also full of antioxidants and omega 3 and may assist with cholesterol levels. They have anti-inflammatory properties and may assist with insulin resistance. They contain protein, calcium, phosphorus, iron, potassium, manganese, zinc, copper, vitamins A and D, Omega 3 and 6. They work as a natural appetite suppressant.

Chicken – organic or free range only.

On this one it does make a difference to pick organic where possible. With its high protein content chicken is a food that reaches across the nutritional spectrum. Naturally low in fat and versatile, it really does deserve a place on the superfoods list. In addition to being a prime source of protein chicken contains amino acids , vitamins B1, B2, B3, B5, B6, B12, B9, B7, choline, zinc, copper, phosphorus, magnesium, and iron.

Chilli peppers

Acting as an anti-inflammatory in line with other capsicums, chillies may assist with pain from arthritis and psoriasis. They are also considered useful in relation to reduction of blood cholesterol and can lower the resting heart rate. Considered as a useful remedy for the symptoms of colds is does actually stimulate secretions that help clear mucus from your stuffed up nose or congested lungs. They contain Vitamins E, A, B6, K, B3, B2, potassium, fibre, copper, manganese and iron.

Cranberries

Cranberry juice is best known for its urinary tract health properties as it acts as a barrier for bacteria attaching itself to the tract and the stomach lining itself. More research is underway and their health properties seem to be increasing as research continues. They contain vitamins C, E, K fibre, manganese, copper and B5.

Dark chocolate

Chocolate lovers, finally some good news! Full of monounsaturated fatty acids, dark chocolate can stimulate CCK and make you feel fuller for longer. These fatty acids along with the flavonols in dark chocolate that can assist in keeping healthy blood pressure and generally be all; round heart friendly. Don't go too crazy but it is loaded with antioxidants so may assist in combating certain cell damage, some cancers and help your skin stay looking good. It contains vitamins A, C, K, B12, B2, B5, calcium, phosphorus, selenium, copper, potassium, magnesium, and iron. (impressive!)

Eggs

Eggs were demonised a few years ago in relation to their cholesterol content but this has since proved to have no effect on your own cholesterol. High in protein and omega 3 and something that will fill you up until lunch, eggs are an excellent breakfast food. They contain some trace elements that are difficult to get from other foods. They are considered a source of pure protein and are high in omega 3 but also contain vitamins A, D, B1, B2, B3, B5, B6, B12, choline, calcium, zinc, iron, copper, manganese, B7, selenium, molybdenum, iodine, B5, carotenoids phosphorus and folic acid.

Flaxseeds/ Linseeds

When you think of omega 3 oils you tend to look towards eggs and fish but weight for weight flaxseeds/linseeds contain almost as much omega 3. These very small seeds also have more antioxidant polyphenols than blueberries and are heart healthy, as they assist with cholesterol levels and are being researched in relation to their potential in relation to insulin resistance. They have anti-carcinogenic benefits are anti-inflammatory, assist digestive health and can even assist with peri and post-menopausal symptoms. They are high in omega 3 fats and also contain vitamins B1, copper, manganese, fibre, magnesium, selenium, and phosphorus.

Garlic

Entire books have been written on the subject of garlic and its healthful and medicinal properties. Known as a blood pressure regulator and heart friendly garlic is also an antiviral and has anti-inflammatory properties. It contains, in addition to is numerous constituents that reduce risk of oxidative stress Vitamins B1, B6, C, calcium, selenium, copper and manganese.

Ginger

Boosting your immune system and settling your stomach ginger really has its place with the super foods. It contains a very strong anti-inflammatory that can assist osteoarthritis and similar conditions. It is being researched in relation to its cancer anti – tumour properties. It can promote healthy sweating and alleviate some symptoms of colds and viral infections. It contains Vitamins C, magnesium, potassium, copper, B9, choline, calcium, and phosphorus

Grapefruit (pink or red)

Every time you pick up a diet sheet grapefruit are thrust at you from all directions! There is a good reason for this though. This is so nutrient dense and rich in antioxidants that it has been recognised for many years as a super food. One of its attributes can actually lower insulin and directly assist in weight loss. It has been linked to reduction in likelihood of prostate cancer; it may reduce inflammatory diseases such as arthritis; Limonoids in grapefruit may assist in eliminating toxins from the body whilst also helping to fight cancers of the mouth stomach and colon. Like apples, they contain pectin which assists in the lowering of cholesterol. They contain Vitamin C, A, B1, B7, B5, potassium, copper and fibre

Green tea

So good for you it features in every modern eating regime intending to increase health. Least processed of all the teas it contains the most antioxidant properties. Green tea is alleged to boost weight loss, reduce cholesterol, combat cardiovascular disease, and prevent cancer and Alzheimer's disease.

Lentils

Rich in dietary fibre to keep you digestive tract happy and packing a serious nutritional punch. These little legumes assist in lowering cholesterol, reducing the risk of heart disease; They can assist in regulating blood sugar and can reduce your risk of diabetes. They contain fibre, copper, vitamins B1, B6, B9, B5, B7, potassium, zinc, protein, iron, manganese, phosphorus and molybdenum.

Miso

Tasty (when you get used to it) and a very handy snack soup as it comes in paste form I use miso soup base as something to grab when I am a little hungry but not ready for a meal. It is quite high in sodium but in a format that does not seem to negatively affect blood pressure. Miso is high in antioxidants, good for your digestive tract, has anti-inflammatory and anti-cancer benefits and contains vitamins K and B2, manganese, copper, protein, choline, omega 3 zinc and phosphorus.

Olive Oil

So what is the secret of the Mediterranean diet? Opinion seems to indicate the olive oil! With an extensive list of phytonutrients including the all-important polyphenols that act as antioxidants and anti-inflammatory properties it is not surprising to hear it also has cardiovascular and digestive health benefits. It also lowers your risk of certain cancers. In addition to the amazing polyphenol content it also contains choline, vitamins E and K, calcium, iron and potassium but it is the omega 3 and 6 fatty acid content that puts it up with the top healthy foods.

Onions

A staple of many meals these not only add flavour but also assists in protecting you from some cancers, may help lower cholesterol, assist with red blood cells and bone density in post-menopausal women and have anti-inflammatory properties. They contain biotin, manganese, copper, vitamin B6, B7, B9 and C, potassium and phosphorus.

Pineapple

Anti-inflammatory, antioxidant, and can assist eye health. An all-round asset to health. It contains vitamins B1, B5, B6, B9, C, copper and manganese.

Pine Nuts

These are so incredibly good for you it is worth including them in you eating plan although – watch out for the high calories. On the up side they are nutritionally dense and contain pineolenic acid (remember oleic acid from the avocadoes?) this stimulates production of CCK and act as a natural appetite suppressant. They contain calcium, fibre, iron, magnesium, manganese, choline, phosphorus, selenium, zinc and vitamins A, C, E, K, B1, B2, B3, B5, B6 and B9.

Quinoa (*pronounced 'keen wa' apparently*)

Nutritionally superior to most grain this, now readily available, grain has both antioxidant and anti-inflammatory properties as well as containing omega 3 and omega 6. It has enough fibre to keep your digestion happy but also is a very good source of protein. It contains manganese, phosphorus, copper, magnesium, zinc, vitamins B9 and E. In addition it has a good amount of oleic acid which stimulates CCK and can help you feel fuller for longer.

Raspberries

Are good for you and tasty and an asset to weight maintenance. Some of the phytonutrients, especially one known as rheosmin, sometimes called raspberry ketone. Raspberries have both antioxidant and anti-aging properties and also are linked to anti-cancer benefits. They contain vitamins C, K, E, B9, B7, B5, potassium, omega 3, magnesium and manganese.

Sage

I have added sage here because it has a specific benefit but you should check before adding it to you eating plan as it can have adverse effect on certain conditions and medications if you have a lot of it. It is packed with antioxidants and has an anti-inflammatory affect. It has a very specific benefit to brain function and is being researched in relation to Alzheimer's and memory loss. It contains vitamins C and K, potassium, manganese

Salmon

Best known for omega 3 related benefits but more recently researched for the benefits of its bioactive peptides which may support not only joint cartilage but also increase insulin effectiveness and assist in controlling digestive tract inflammation. Omega 3 cardiovascular benefits are well documented but now a link between brain function and omega 3 is being suggested. Salmon is joint friendly due to its anti-inflammatory benefits and also assists in protecting the eyes. It has some anti-carcinogenic properties. It contains vitamins B6, B12, D, B3, selenium, omega 3, choline, B5, potassium and B7.

Sardines

Rich in omega 3 and packed with heart and bone friendly vitamins sardines are a good addition to this list. They contain vitamins B2, B3, B12, D, and Omega 3, phosphorus, selenium, copper, calcium and choline.

Soy Beans/ Endame Beans

Soy beans make a considerable contribution nutritionally like all legumes. Unlike many they have a high protein content and contain some of the more unusual peptides that are linked to lower blood pressure, blood sugar control and can even be beneficial to the immune system. Having a beneficial effect on cholesterol and potential offering cardiovascular support they also have be suggested to have anti-carcinogenic properties. Soy beans can have a beneficial effect on bone health and type two diabetes. They contain vitamin K, B2, C, protein, omega 3 oils, fibre, iron, magnesium, molybdenum, copper, manganese, phosphorus and potassium.

Spinach

Is good for you – no surprise there, then! Anti-cancer and anti-inflammatory with loads of vitamin K to help your bones – Popeye was not far wrong. It has a massive nutritional content including vitamins A,B1, B2, B5, B6, B9, selenium, omega 3, choline, zinc, protein, potassium, phosphorus, calcium, copper, iron, are you bored yet, magnesium, and manganese.

Sweet Potatoes.

Excellent source of beta carotene and antioxidants they have anti-inflammatory properties and can assist with blood sugar regulation. They contain vitamins A, C, B6, B3, B1, B2, phosphorus, potassium, fibre, copper, manganese, B5 and B7.

Tomatoes

Packed full of nutrients tomatoes provide cardiovascular support , anti-cancer benefits and have more recently linked to reducing the likelihood of neurological issues such as Alzheimer's. They have a very high concentrate of antioxidants and phytonutrients and can support bone health especially in peri-menopausal and menopausal women. They contain vitamins B1, B6, B3, A, E, C, K, and B7, molybdenum, copper, potassium, fibre, B9, manganese, phosphorus, magnesium, chromium, B5, choline, zinc and iron.

Tuna

Anti-oxidant, anti-inflammatory, anti-cancer and a good source of lean protein Tuna is a beneficial addition to any eating plan. Also containing omega 3 it is heart and brain friendly as well. It contains protein, selenium, vitamins B3, B6, B12, D, B1, and B2, magnesium, choline and phosphorus.

Watercress

It is amazing. It contains more vitamin C than oranges, more calcium than milk and more iron than spinach. It is anti-inflammatory, anti-cancer; helps maintain the blood, high in fibre and a good source of iodine. It contains vitamins A, C, B1, B6 and K along with calcium, iron, magnesium, potassium, manganese, choline, zinc, phosphorus, and copper. It has been reputed to have an aphrodisiac effect too

The 'Rumour has it' Bit

I am not stating that all this research into what is good for you in what way is gospel truth– I just thought it might be handy to have an easy list of the current suggested benefits of certain foods. If you discover any more I have left a few rows for you to add your own or pop an extra 'x' in any that you discover have additional benefits
This is just a brief summary of what is linked to which benefit. So here goes.

Column values
1. Heart and blood pressure
2. Cancer
3. Digestion
4. Cholesterol
5. Blood sugar
6. Kidneys and Liver
7. Skin
8. Joints
9. Weight
10. Brain Function

	1	2	3	4	5	6	7	8	9	10
Almonds	X		X	X			X	X	X	X
Apples			X	X	X	X	X		X	
Apricots	X						X			
Asparagus	X	X	X	X	X	X		X	X	
Avocados	X	X	X	X				X	X	
Bananas	X		X							
Beetroot	X	X			X	X	X		X	X
Bell peppers		X		X		X	X	X	X	
Black beans		X								
Blueberries	X	X		X	X		X	X	X	X
Brazil nuts		X								X
Broccoli	X	X	X	X			X		X	

	1	2	3	4	5	6	7	8	9	10
Brown rice		X	X	X	X					
Cauliflower	X	X	X			X		X	X	
Chia Seeds										
Chillies	X			X				X	X	
Cherries	X	X	X		X	X	X	X	X	
Cranberries		X	X				X		X	
Dark chocolate	X	X	X				X		X	
Garlic	X				X	X		X		
Ginger			X				X	X	X	
Grapefruit		X		X	X			X	X	
Green tea	X	X	X	X			X	X	X	X
Linseed/ Flaxseed	X	X	X	X			X	X	X	
Lentils	X	X	X	X	X				X	
Miso	X	X	X							X
Olive Oil	X	X	X	X		X	X	X		X
Onion	X	X		X	X	X		X		
Pineapple		X		X				X		
Pine nuts	X	X		X			X	X		X
Quinoa	X	X	X	X	X			X	X	
Salmon	X	X	X	X			X	X	X	X
Sardines										X
Soy beans	X	X	X	X			X	X	X	X
Sweet potato			X		X			X	X	
Tomato	X	X		X			X	X	X	X
Tuna	X	X	X	X				X		X
Watercress	X	X	X	X	X	X	X	X	X	X

The 'A Few Small Changes' bit

If you never want to diet again, and I certainly don't, you do need to think about making a few small changes.

You may already be looking at the super foods bit and thinking you might want to include a few in the way you eat but there are a few basic simple changes that may help you reduce in size and weight without too much impact. You have a choice – you can choose to change and be choosey or choose to be chubby!

1. **Change from sugar to stevia.**
   To start with it may taste a little different but you will become accustomed to it. It is not like the old fashioned sweeteners – no bitter aftertaste. Your simple choice is to change this one little thing for quite a large impact.

2. **Change from your normal bread to soya and linseed bread.**
   It is a little dearer but very satisfying, generally much healthier and linseed has so many healthy properties that assist in appetite suppression that you should at least try it for a week

3. **Change from potatoes to sweet potatoes**
   They are low GI and lower carbohydrate than but at least as satisfying as regular potatoes. Faster to cook so they lose less nutrients by the time you put them on your plate. Great roasted and in soups and turned into chips they make a great accompaniment to most dishes

4. **Eat half a pink or red grapefruit each day or at least each second day**.
   Due to all its wonderful qualities adding half a pink or red grapefruit each day can actually assist you weight reduction to the cost of half a pound a week. Burn off that belly with this simple step.

5. **Drink more water**
   Assists in eliminating toxins; improves your skin; aids concentration; loves your liver; reduces your appetite. Where is the bad?

6. **Drink Green Tea**
   Appetite suppressing and an all-round good guy – this is its third mention in the book so far.

7. **Get nutty**
   Swap out your unhealthy snacks for almonds or another nut. Filling and a healthy alternative, there is a nut out there for you. Just try them all until you find one you like. Be a little conscious that some are quite high in calories etc so don't go completely crazy but they have a longer 'fullness factor' than sugar based snacks and are much more beneficial health wise.

8. **Change from pasta and noodles to either low carb pasta or shiratake noodles and pasta.**
   Pasta is great if you are an athlete otherwise it is not great staple food for those wanting to gain and retain their perfect shape.

9. **Get those greens tasting good**
   Learn to do something interesting with asparagus and broccoli (stir fried in sesame oil with oyster sauce?) then try to eat it more regularly.

10. **Avoid diet/low fat foods unless you read the package first**
    They are usually not as good as they should be (with some exceptions)

The 'What about diets?' bit.

They don't work – not in the long term.
If they did the diet industry would not be worth £2 billion and growing.
They certainly help you lose pounds – straight out of your pocket.
Absolutely it is possible to get a short term burst of weight reduction. If you want to briefly give yourself the buzz of quick inch reduction – go for it.
Of course it will be back and you will feel like you have failed but maybe if you try one of the major diet types – if there are any you have not already tried – you will remind yourself how they are quick but not sustainable.
The major players in the industry at the moment are based on the below methodologies

Calorie controlled
Rapid weight loss can be motivating but it is unsustainable – very low calorie diets will have short term results that are impressive but are hard to sustain over a long period.

Low Fat
Can reduce weight quickly and feel quite healthy except for the fact that many low fat foods are higher in carbohydrates. Low fat diets are not sustainable over a long period and it is important to remember that many fats contain essential nutrients that you will be missing in a low fat diet

Low carbohydrate.
Reducing carbohydrates in a safe and healthy way will have a very impressive result. A very low carb diet can lead to constipation, bad breath and nutritional deficiency if you avoid some high carb food groups like fruit. Reducing your carbs does tend to lead to reducing you processed food intake and this is both effective and healthy – as long as you are careful.

Weekly fasting (5/2)
The 5:2 is a simple way to reduce calorie intake. There are lots of versions of this diet, with some less safe than others. It is important to avoid nutritional deficiencies, dehydration and overeating on non-fast days.

Food combining / Alkaline Diet
Limiting you food groups in relation to the amount of time food takes to digest and how the acid and alkaline in your stomach work with each other can assist your digestion in functioning efficiently and also assist in reducing your weight and size. Most these eating plans offer some very sensible eating choices but do mean that you need to be fully aware of every food choice and recipe.

High Fibre
High fibre diets are also working with your digestive system and concentrate on making you feel fuller for longer by using high fibre menus and meal replacements. A bit too boring to sustain (just my opinion as a foodie) although the do have same very good overall health benefits.

Meal replacement diets
Replacing real tasty nutritious inexpensive food with expensive stuff that is almost but not quite food – I have nothing good to say about these unsustainable short term fixes – I like food to be ...food. If you want to go down that road, look them up yourself.

In the next few pages are diet plans.
Look at them as an example of what is out there.

If you want to use any of them, do – you will just prove to yourself that you can only achieve sustainable weight reduction by following the rules in this book not limiting yourself to some restrictive eating plan.

What follows are diets.

What you are aiming to do is not ever diet again but I know you want to at least see some form of eating plan in a 'diet' book Feel free to flirt with them all then come back to me when you are done.
Then you can follow the rules, not diet and experiment with some of the awesome recipes toward the end of the book.

For any *diet* plan a good all round vitamin supplement is advised to ensure all nutritional needs are met. It never hurts to use some psyllium husk capsules and these keep things 'moving'. Plus – Check with your doctor before you go on ANY diet. Ensure you take enough water. Ice water has a thermogenic effect. Green tea stimulates CCK.

So, if you feel you must do it here are some of the current trends.

Calorie controlled diet examples

Your body requires a deficit of 3500 calories to reduce by one pound. By reducing your calorific intake you will lose weight. (Not much fun though)

Example of a 1000 calorie menu – diets this low in calories should not be followed for more than four or five days. Your body starts to go into starvation mode and will want to conserve energy and store as much excess as it can.

Breakfast example

Half a grapefruit
1 boiled egg
1 slice wholegrain toast (scraped with butter)
Tea or coffee (no milk)

Lunch example

2 slices of cold chicken/ turkey (no skin) or lean beef.
Large green salad mixing rocket, watercress, lettuce, cucumber
6 cherry tomatoes
1 slice wholegrain toast (no butter)
Tea or coffee (no milk)

Dinner example

125grams grilled fish or 150 grams of chicken (no skin)
1 cup of steamed broccoli
1 cup of steamed cauliflower
Tea or coffee

You may season with salt and pepper only.
Drink a large glass of water before every meal
No sugar or milk
Teas may be standard or herbal.
You may drink unlimited herbal teas.

Example of a 1500 calorie diet

Breakfast example

Toast & boiled egg

2 slices of wholegrain bread toasted and spread with 2 teaspoon low fat spread.
One boiled egg
Tea or coffee
1 banana

Lunch example

Salmon salad sandwich with fruit

Two slices of granary bread filled with 120grams salmon mixed with one tablespoon of lower fat mayonnaise and plenty of mixed salad.
1 low fat yoghurt
Tea or coffee

Snack example

Cottage cheese with fruit

120grams of cottage cheese and two mandarins and up to ten grapes

Dinner example

Pasta salad with broccoli and tomatoes.

75grams of pasta (or twice that if you use eat water pasta)
90 grams of broccoli (steamed)
6 cherry tomatoes
20 grams of flaked almonds

Dress with two tablespoons of low fat yoghurt, three teaspoons
of pesto, salt and black pepper, fresh parsley or basil
Tea or coffee

No sugar but a quarter of a pint of skimmed milk per day
Drink a large glass of water before every meal
Teas may be standard or herbal.
You may drink unlimited herbal teas.

Low fat diet example

Quite strict and watch out for the extra carbs in anything calling itself low fat. Take a good vitamin supplement if you try this to ensure you have adequate fat soluble vitamins included.

Breakfast example

Toast with marmalade and fruit

Two slices wholemeal toast
Two teaspoons of low-fat spread and marmalade.
A bowl of raspberries.

Lunch example

Turkey sandwich, mousse and fruit

Two slices wholemeal bread filled with 125 grams of wafer-thin turkey, two teaspoons of cranberry sauce and salad. One pot low-fat mousse any flavour and a mandarin or kiwi fruit.

Dinner example

Roast beef and Yorkshire pud followed by fruit salad

Three thin slices lean roast beef with one small ready-made Yorkshire pudding, five new potatoes boiled in their skins, a small portion of green vegetables, a teaspoon of horseradish sauce and fat-free gravy.

A bowl of fresh fruit salad with a tablespoon of single cream.

Low carbohydrate diet example

Many people still believe that eating fat makes you fat but now it is understood that your body store excess carbohydrates as fat.

Your body finds carbohydrate as its most easily accessible form of fuel. Once you reduce the carbohydrates in you regime your body starts to look for other fuel and quickly starts to use you fat stores as fuel. Your body will crave carbohydrates for a few days until it adapts. You are aiming for less than 80grams of carbohydrate each day. (Your breath will be quite unpleasant too)

You may eat freely

Meat Beef, lamb, pork, chicken and others.

Fish Salmon, trout, haddock and any others.

Eggs All

Vegetables Spinach, broccoli, cauliflower, and all non starchy vegetables

Nuts and Seeds Almonds, walnuts, sunflower seeds, flax.

High-Fat Dairy Cheese, butter, heavy cream, yogurt.

Fats and Oils Coconut oil, butter, lard, olive oil and cod fish liver oil.

Sweeteners Stevia

Noodles Shiratake noodles only –no carbs – almost no calories

In moderation

Fruits Apples, oranges, pears, blueberries, strawberries.

Tubers Sweet potatoes and butternut squash

Very carefully

Non-gluten grains Brown rice, oats, quinoa

Legumes Lentils, black beans, pinto beans.

Dark Chocolate 70% cocoa or higher.

Wine Choose dry wines – red is better

You may not eat under any circumstance

Breads pasta and cakes Bread, cake, biscuits, pasta, noodles, crackers

Sugar based products Soft drinks, fruit juices, sweeties, ice cream and you can guess the others

Gluten Grains Wheat, spelt, barley and rye.

Trans Fats Hydrogenated or partially hydrogenated oils.

Vegetable Oils Sunflower, grape seed, corn oil

Artificial Sweeteners Aspartame, Saccharin, Sucralose

Anything with 'diet' or 'low fat' on it

Breakfast examples

Bacon and eggs Or Cheese omelette
Tea or coffee

Lunch examples

Chicken salad with loads of chicken with the salad dressed with olive oil Or Salmon with steamed vegetables
Tea or coffee

Dinner examples

Steak and vegetables Or Chicken stir fried with onion, garlic, broccoli, shiratake noodles soy sauce
Sugar free jelly
Large glass of water or wine

Nothing processed
Drink a large glass of water before each meal.

Intermittent fasting diet (5/2)

Eat normally for five days each week
For two days each week eat no more than five hundred calories for women or six hundred for men. You really, really need to up your liquid intake. Herbal teas are good green tea is better. Do not over exert yourself on your fast days.

Five hundred calorie day menu examples
Day One

Breakfast

Two eggs – hard boiled/soft boiled/poached/scrambled – no added fat
Green tea (140 cals)

Lunch

100 grams chicken breast with salad of mixed leaves
(as much as you can eat in one sitting)
5 cherry tomatoes
Green tea (140)

Dinner

Stir fried shiratake noodles with 150 grams chicken breast, one spring onion, garlic, six mushrooms, grated fresh ginger, a dash of soy sauce, chillies (optional) half a teaspoon of sesame oil .
Green tea (210)
Day total 490

Day Two
Breakfast

Two eggs – hard boiled/soft boiled/poached/scrambled – no added fat
Green tea (140)

Lunch

120 grams sliced turkey breast with salad of mixed leaves
(as much as you can eat in one sitting.) and 5 cherry tomatoes
Green tea (140)

Dinner

Eat water pasta shapes cooked with 100 grams lean ham half an onion, garlic, six mushrooms, two table spoons of chopped tomatoes and any herbs you wish to add.(220)
Green tea
Day total 500

Food Combining/Alkaline Diet

Food combining separates foods into three main categories of which only specific combinations are allowed. The food combining diet looks at the chemical imbalance within the digestive tract. It addresses the different rate at which your body digests food and how the wrong combinations reduce the efficiency of your body's digestive process. If there is an accumulation of acid from digestion and metabolism in amounts greater than you can eliminate it lowers your alkaline reserve which can cause autointoxication. Effectively your body is poisoning itself.

So this food combining diet is designed to ensure these conditions do not happen and therefore the body should maintain it's natural chemical balances.

Protein	Neutral	Carbohydrate
Meat	Non starchy vegetables	Potatoes
Poultry	Salad vegetables	Bread
Cheese	Seeds	Cakes
Eggs	Nuts	Biscuits
Fish	Herbs	Pasta
Soya beans	Butter	Oats
Yoghurt	Olive Oil	Rice
Tofu	Shiratake Noodles	Sugar (in any form)

From the above categories you may eat any combination of protein and neutral or any combination of carbohydrate and neutral. At no time may you combine carbohydrate and protein. Whilst you are advised to use fresh rather than processed food any processed food should have the ingredients list thoroughly checked to ensure the combination rules are not broken.

The 'Eating for specific benefits' bit

If you are embarking on the new long term slightly healthier you, you might want to try some of these detoxes to give your organs a bit of a once over. Or you might want to try them sometime down the line – or even not at all. But here they are; One for your liver; one for your kidneys; one for your colon. Do make sure that you are healthy enough to try them and also that none of the ingredients clash with or reduce the effect of any medicine you are taking. Check with your doctor if you have any health issues as there is no point trying to do something healthy and making yourself ill.

The 'Love your liver' detox smoothies

Your liver is doing a very important job but can accumulate a lot of toxins on the way
It can be negatively affected by pollution in the air and water and in our foods. It can have difficulty with pesticides in the food chain, artificial additives, preservatives, sweeteners, medicines, and processed foods.

When it is working ok it regulates your temperature, stores certain vitamins maintains blood sugar levels very importantly removes many toxins and stops them getting into your blood. It also makes bile to help break stuff down into what your body needs amongst other jobs.

It is so taken for granted as it removes the goodness from our food and turns the toxins etc into waste matter that we mostly don't realise what a great job it is doing.

A healthy liver diet reduces the strain on your liver. Looking after your liver will increase your overall health and means that with your body, metabolism and digestion working properly maintaining your ideal size and weight becomes easier.

These detoxes should be handled with care as they can have quite a strong reaction on your system. Short term discomfort for long term gain, as it were. Any advantage you can get that means you do not have to diet is an advantage that is worth taking.

So here goes – and I will not tell you this will taste particularly nice but it will make you feel like you are really doing something for your lovely liver.

Liver cleansing smoothie 1

- 300 ml of cranberry juice
- 1 large red grapefruit (peeled)
- 20 blueberries (fresh or frozen)
- 2 tablespoons of olive oil
- 1 small probiotic drink (Yakult or similar)
- 1 clove of garlic
- About 2 inches of ginger – grated
- The juice of 1 lemon
- 25 grams of linseeds/ flaxseeds
- A small fresh chilli if you can face it (deseed it unless you want a real burn)
- A handful of spinach

Into the blender and make a great big smelly smoothie. Make sure no one can take a photo of your face when you drink it. It makes a big batch and will take a while to drink but will make you feel full. On this occasion give yourself permission NOT to stop drinking when you have had enough! It takes me about half an hour to get through it.

Don't eat or drink anything else for the next two to three hours – ideally do this on a day when you go lie down, read a book and take it easy. If fact you could give yourself a 'spa' day with face pack and hair conditioner mask – try those funky foot moisturizing socks (available in pound world)...... or sit and play your XBOX or PS for a few hours

After three hours feel free to eat as much fresh clean food as you like – salads, veggie soup (see recipes) broccoli, cauliflower, asparagus etc – keep it bland for today with the exception of ground black pepper and drink at least a litre and a half of cold water. If you want a hot drink – get the green tea on.

This is pretty awesome for your liver but too strong to do more than once every three months or so – if you can face it again. It does help enhance you toxin removal – a polite way of saying at some point in the next 24 hours you will feel really clean.

Liver cleansing smoothie 2

- Juice of 2 lemons
- 1 large red grapefruit
- 300mls of no added sugar cranberry juice drink
- 2 tablespoon extra virgin olive oil
- 1 Yakult or similar
- 2 cloves of garlic
- 1 vacuum packed cooked beetroot
- 2 inches of grated fresh ginger root
- 1 medium red chili – deseeded if you do not want a burn.

Everything into your jug blender or smoothie maker and blend until smooth enough to drink. You can add more water if it is still too gloopy for your liking.

Try not to eat or drink for two or three hours and keep it light and natural for the rest of the day. Take it easy on yourself again and rest up a bit to give your body a real treat.

This is also too strong to do too often. Every couple of months maybe?

The downside of any detoxifying smoothie or even soup is that it does eliminate toxins – sometimes a bit quickly - so a dodgy tummy is not at all unlikely. You may also get a bit gassy but it is all in a good cause.

For a light and generally more user friendly helping hand to your liver you could just make up the following nice and healthy juice drink which will help burn fat, suppress your appetite and help your body work better.

Generally healthy juice drink.

- 300mls cranberry juice – or no added juice drink
- 1 litre of water
- Juice of 2 lemons
- 300mls orange juice – not from concentrate
- ½ teaspoon cinnamon powder
- 1 teaspoon Tabasco
- 2 teaspoon stevia – or honey – to taste
- 1 tablespoon ground flaxseed or chia seeds

Mix well in a jug blender and drink at regular intervals throughout your day, all day, and any day.

Big list of liver friendly things

broccoli	asparagus	kale	cabbage
Spinach	rocket	watercress	beetroot
cauliflower	onions	mangos	grapefruit
lemons	papaya	pears	apples
brown rice	oatmeal	rye	barley
lentils	garbanzo beans	kidney beans	garlic
nutmeg	cinnamon	ginger	all nuts
seeds	olive oil	flax seed oil	chili

Add them to your eating – if you have not already.

The 'kiss your kidneys' detox smoothie.

You kidneys also flush waste products from your system and as such can also appreciate the occasional cleanse. There is a fair bit of Parsley in this and parsley can be a bit strong on your system so once again, check before you give this a go. Do not have this if you are pregnant.
It tastes considerably better than the liver detox smoothie!

- 2 large carrots
- 2 sticks of celery
- 1 beetroot (vacuum packed or fresh but not pickled)
- ½ a cucumber
- Juice of 1 lemon
- ½ ounce of parsley
- 20 blueberries (fresh or frozen)
- 300 ml of cranberry juice.

Blend together and drink
As with the liver day – give it a couple of hours before eating but drink plenty of cold water and green tea.
This is also too strong to do more than once every couple of weeks.

The 'cuddle your colon' detox smoothies and soup

Over looked and underappreciated your colon – aka large intestine – is probably as long as you are tall as it is on average between five and six feet long. Food that is digesting can spend up to ninety percent of its time in the colon getting all its goodness and juice squeezed out as it travels through your digestive system on a journey that can take up to three days.

Some bits can hang around longer than is ideal but a good level of fibre in your eating habits can not only help keep everything moving but also helps avoid bladder and kidney infections, thrush, bad breath, body odour, abdominal cramps as well as constipation. A healthy colon efficiently eliminates toxins. An unhealthy colon allows toxins to back up into the liver and bloodstream, polluting the entire system – by which I mean your entire body.

So your poor old colon is trying very hard to keep us healthy but with the amount of processed, low fibre food in our modern diet colons are struggling and quickly becoming one of the most common places to contract cancer.

A bit of extra help now and again can assist in maintaining colon health and a healthy rate of peristalsis. This is the squeezing motion that the colon uses to move food through its length. Fibre is particularly important in this function. The other health issue can be that your body does not produce as many digestive enzymes as you get older – which explains why many people are more prone to indigestion as they mature.
Salads, and any raw vegetables, provide digestive enzymes that can top up the body's supply and help colon health.
Water– once again drinking enough water, around two litres of liquid a day, will help you colon as well as your kidneys and liver.
Lastly feed your friendly bacteria. Probiotics are rumoured to assist in digestive health and foods high in inulin feed the bacteria and assist in healthy digestion.

Apart from the obvious benefits of a healthy colon, getting your digestion sorted out will improve your overall health and you will see visible improvements in your skin condition. Two to three poops a day would indicate your colon is doing a fine job.

Here are a couple of colon detox smoothies and a soup that should get everything moving – you can have one of these every day if you like. It should improve your general health.

Colon Smoothie 1

- 20 blueberries (fresh or frozen)
- 10 raspberries (fresh or frozen)
- Half a cucumber
- Two tablespoons of oat bran
- 1 small probiotic drink (e.g. yakult)
- A handful of spinach leaves or rocket.
- 300mls of almond milk or apple juice
- 2 tablespoons of linseeds/chia seeds
- 1 medium carrot (chopped smallish before blending)

A few ice cubes or a little chilled water if you want it a little more liquid
Blend and enjoy

I like mine about mid morning instead of a snack.
I will not go into details as to exactly what you should expect – it's a colon cleanse use your imagination - but I would avoid long journeys with no facilities for 24 hours...........

Colon smoothie 2

- 300mls of cranberry juice drink – no added sugar
- 1 tin of pineapple in juice or about half a fresh pineapple peeled etc.
- 1 cucumber – skin on I'm afraid
- 200 grams kale shredded
- juice of one lemon, squeezed
- ½ an inch of ginger grated
- 1 bunch of mint

Blend until smooth enough to drink – add more water if you like.

Colon smoothie 3

- 300mls almond milk or coconut water
- 1 tablespoon linseed (flaxseed) or chia seeds or both
- About 20 blueberries – fresh or frozen
- ½ a banana
- About 10 raspberries
- A mango – I use about ten frozen pieces as they are a pain to peel etc

Blend and enjoy (adding more liquid if you need to)

I like to make a lot of this one to drink throughout the day each time I fancy a snack

Colon cleanse soup.

- 2 onions
- 1 tablespoon of olive oil
- 2 garlic cloves
- 2 celery stalks
- 1 fennel bulb with all it's bits
- 10 mushrooms
- 1 Savoy cabbage
- 2tablespoons of paprika
- 8 sprigs parsley
- A handful of sage leaves
- 2 teaspoons of caraway seeds
- About 2 pints of vegetable stock – made up as per instructions
- As much ground black pepper as you like

1. Heat the oil in a large stock/soup pan
2. Chop the onion, garlic, celery, fennel, and fry off for a few minutes.
3. Chop and add the mushrooms and fry stirring quickly for a few minutes more – if it seems a bit dry add a little stock
4. Add the herbs and seasoning – don't be limited by the recipe if you have a favorite herb
5. Add the stock and bring to a boil then simmer until all the veggies are soft.
6. Add more stock if you like a looser texture.
7. Scoop about 2/3 of the veggies into a blender and puree
8. Re add this to the soup to thicken.
9. Bring back to a bubble and serve piping hot with some soya and linseed toast.

The 'Going a step further with some really healthy recipes' bit

Remember – you are NOT on a diet but you are just making a few healthy choices. The rules still apply

Eat only when you are hungry
Eat slowly and mindfully
Stop when you have had enough.

Remembering that you don't want to diet but recognising that you realise by now that if you eat the sort of food that helps your body be very very healthy then you will lose more weight as your body is working at its optimum level.
Mostly sometimes you want to eat something nice, sometimes you want to eat something nice that is also good for you. For those days when you are feeling like being really really healthy – the following recipes are healthy and tasty – not, unfortunately, in a smothered in butter way but quite tasty anyway.

I have listed the calories for some – sorry about that but sometimes it is useful to know that some things can taste good and not be hugely bad for you.
The benefits of eating well and using the healthier option are extensive you will find that you:

> Burn fat more easily
> Increase your energy levels
> Reduce your hunger pangs
> Detox your system – kidneys, liver and colon – when it works better you feel better.
> Make you feel better by stabilising your blood sugar
> Improve circulation
> Help your joints with anti inflammatory properties
> Lower your cholesterol levels
> Help your brain function

> Relieve depression, anxiety and stress
> Help achieve a good sleep pattern
> Make you glow with healthy skin, nails and hair
> Generally feel very very good.

Remember you ARE NOT DIETING.

A few small changes will start to achieve this but here is a bit of hard core healthy for those days you want to be ultra-good to yourself.

Try a day like this

- Breakfast: 2 scrambled eggs on a slice of Soya and Linseed toast, mushrooms poached in a teaspoon of butter and 3 tablespoons of water – bubble these until the water has gone and they sizzle.
- A big cup of green tea and a half litre of water with the juice half a lemon.

- Snack: A plain yogurt and an orange

- Lunch: salad of rocket, watercress, spinach, Swiss chard– chuck in some basil and parsley if you fancy it – any fresh green herb is good. (As much green as you want); half an avocado, beetroot and spring onion salad on the side; 6 oz of lean protein – chicken/salmon/ turkey/ smoked salmon. Dress with a little olive oil and red wine vinegar, black pepper and low salt

- Green tea and a large glass of water.

- Snack: An apple and a dozen cherries and 10 unsalted almonds.

- Dinner: as much broccoli and cauliflower as you want. (Try dry frying it with garlic and black pepper after it is cooked – use half tsp olive oil for better flavor) and 8 oz. of protein, as for lunch. Green Tea, large glass of water.

- Before Bed – herbal/night time tea – (heath and heather night time tea is good)

If you get hungry at any time have another dozen cherries or another 10 almonds.

Dishes under 300 calories

Really good prawns

Serves 1 – double for 2

- 2teaspoon olive oil
- 1 clove garlic, crushed
- ½ teaspoon smoked paprika
- 10 mushrooms, sliced thinly
- A handful of flat-leaf parsley sprigs
- 200grams cherry tomatoes
- 2teaspoon Worcester sauce
- ½ tablespoon sun-dried tomato paste
- 10 large raw prawns, peeled, removing the black vein
- Low Salt and ground black pepper
- 1 slice soya and linseed bread, toasted, to serve

Method

1. Heat the oil in a large, shallow pan. Add the garlic, mushrooms and parsley stalks and fry gently for 12-15 mins until tender. Add the cherry tomatoes, wine/port/sherry and tomato paste. Bring to the boil and then bubble until thickening.
2. Put the prawns into the sauce, cook for 2 mins. Turn them and cook for 1-2 mins or until they're pink all over. Season and sprinkle with parsley leaves for serving. Serve with toast

For really good chicken – use chicken breast chopped up quite small instead of prawns.

Tasty Fish Patties

Serves 2

- 400grams (14oz) fish fillet, skinned (any mixture goes)
- 5 tablespoons chopped fresh parsley
- 1 rounded tablespoon of capers, rinsed – you could use finely diced gherkin (dill pickle) if you want a bit of punch
- Juice of a large lemon
- Low salt and ground black pepper
- 1 tablespoon olive oil
- A little flour
- Big dark green salad dressed with a little olive oil and red wine vinegar and black pepper.

Method

1. Finely chop the fish or put it in a food processor and whizz briefly, so that it's still chunky.
2. Add the parsley, capers, lemon zest and seasoning.
3. Squeeze the mixture well in your hand to drain out any water, and then shape into 4 small patties or two larger ones. Put them in the fridge for ten minutes if you have time – they are easier to cook when a little firmer
4. Heat the oil in a pan; sprinkle a little flour on patties.
5. Cook them over a low to medium heat for about 3 mins each side, until browned and just cooked.
6. Serve with green salad and a side of beetroot and onion salad.

Fast Thai curry

Serves 2

- 2 teaspoon toasted sesame oil – you can use olive but the flavour will not be the same.
- 2 chicken breasts chopped up.
- 1 onion
- 1 clove garlic
- 2 tablespoons green curry paste
- 400gram tin light coconut milk
- 1 tablespoon fish sauce
- 1 lime – juice and zest
- 3 spring onions
- 10 mushrooms – oyster if you like but any are good
- 20 sugar snap peas
- Pack of bean sprouts

Method

1. Fry off onion and garlic in the oil.
2. Add chicken and mushrooms. Stir for a few mins until browning
3. Add paste and cook for another minute
4. Pour in coconut milk, fish sauce and lime zest and juice and bring to a simmer
5. Add spring onions, peas and bean sprouts and cook for a further 5 mins or until chicken is cooked – stirring regularly.
6. Serve and enjoy

Pea and mint soup with bacon bits.

Serves 2

- 200grams frozen peas
- 2 leeks – well scrubbed and de-gritted
- 200grams potato scrubbed but not skinned
- 500mls chicken or veggie stock – check for additives
- 150grams no fat yoghurt
- 2 tablespoon chopped fresh mint
- 2 slices prosciutto – remove all fat

Method

1. Chop up the potato and leek and bring them to the boil in the stock and simmer for about 8 minutes.
2. While this is simmering lay the strips of prosciutto in a big frying pan – no oil - and keep an eye on it as you are just trying to crisp it up. When crisp remove and let it cool enough to break it up for sprinkling.
3. to the potatoes and leeks pan, add the peas and cook for another 5 mins
4. Tip into a blender or use a hand blender to whizz until smooth
5. Add the yoghurt
6. Serve and sprinkle with crispy prosciutto bits.

Homemade houmous and veggie dippers

Serves 2

- 400grams can chickpeas, drained
- 1 clove of garlic
- 100grams roasted red pepper – from a jar or roast one yourself.
- 1 tablespoon tahini
- Juice from half a lemon
- 1 tablespoon linseeds or chia seeds
- For dipping
- 1 bell pepper – any colour.
- 2 carrots
- 2 celery sticks
- 2 courgettes.

Method

1. Whizz the chickpeas, garlic, pepper, tahini, linseeds and lemon juice in a processor or blender.
2. Serve in small pots
3. Chop veggies and dip

Salmon and Miso broth

Serves 2

- 18grams instant miso soup
- 2 cloves of garlic finely chopped
- 1 tablespoon white wine vinegar
- 100grams fine stemmed broccoli cut long and thin
- 4 spring onions
- 100grams bean sprouts
- 100grams watercress
- 2 salmon fillets 120 – 140grams each

Method

1. Bring the soup mix, vinegar and garlic to the boil with 500mls of water and simmer for 5 mins
2. Add the broccoli and spring onions, cover and simmer for 5 minutes
3. Stir in the watercress and bean sprouts and top with the salmon.
4. Cook for about 4 or 5 mins until the salmon is cooked through to your taste.
5. Serve and enjoy

Salmon with celeriac gratin

Serves 2

- 400grams celeriac, peeled- about 600grams whole
- 5grams garlic cloves, finely chopped
- 1 tablespoon fresh thyme leaves
- 1 chicken stock cube
- 2 x 100grams skinless salmon fillets
- 1 tablespoon wholegrain mustard
- 300grams green beans

Method

1. Heat oven to 200C/180C fan/gas 6. Slice the celeriac as thinly as you can – quartering it first will help. Find a baking dish that will hold all the celeriac, and then add a layer before scattering with some garlic, thyme and seasoning. Repeat layers, finishing on a celeriac layer.
2. Mix the stock cube with 225ml boiling water, season with nutmeg, then pour over the celeriac. Bake for about 1 hr 15 mins – pressing the celeriac into the dish so that it stays submerged and soaks up the stock – until a skewer poked in goes in easily, and the top is crisp.
3. When the gratin has 15 mins to go, sit the salmon on a baking parchment-lined baking sheet. Mix the mustard with some ground black pepper and a little salt, and brush over the fillets. Bake with the gratin for 12-15 mins until cooked just through.
4. Meanwhile, cook the beans in boiling water until tender, drain well and season. Divide into 2 equal portions along with the gratin, and serve with the salmon.

Singapore noodles

Serves 2

- 100grams skinless chicken breasts, diced
- 50grams raw peeled prawns, chopped
- Juice of half a lemon
- 2 tablespoon medium curry powder
- 300grams cauliflower florets
- 100grams spring onions, whites and greens separately sliced
- 200grams white cabbage, cut into chunks
- 25grams fresh red chillies, finely chopped
- 100grams drained and rinsed shiratake noodles
- 1 tablespoon soy sauce
- ½ teaspoon golden caster sugar
- 5grams coriander leaves (cilantro if you are in the USA)

Method

1. Heat oven to 180C/160C fan/gas 4. Line a baking tray with baking parchment. Mix the lemon juice with ½ tablespoon of the curry powder and toss with the cauliflower on the baking tray. Roast for 25-30 mins until tender and slightly golden.
2. Heat a non-stick wok or frying pan and add the chicken, spring onion whites, cabbage, red chilli, remaining curry powder and a splash of water. Fry, adding splashes of water if it starts sticking or looking dry, until the chicken is cooked through and the cabbage is softening. Add the noodles, prawns, soy sauce and sugar, and fry for another few mins until piping hot and the prawns are cooked. Scatter over the spring onion greens, roasted cauliflower and coriander leaves, and serve.

Chicken gumbo

Serves 2

- 1 tablespoon olive oil
- 250grams skinless, boneless chicken thighs, cut into chunks
- 1 onion, chopped
- 1 green pepper, deseeded and chopped
- 1 celery stick, finely chopped
- 1 garlic clove, finely chopped
- ¼ teaspoon cayenne pepper
- 1 teaspoon smoked paprika
- 1 teaspoon ground cumin
- 1 teaspoon dried thyme
- 1 bay leaf
- 1 heaped tablespoon plain flour
- 250grams tinned chopped tomatoes
- 200ml chicken stock
- 50grams okra, cut into 2cm rounds
- small handful sage, leaves chopped

Method

1. Heat the oil in a large pan over a medium high heat. Add the chicken and cook in batches for about 5 mins to brown all over. Remove the chicken with a slotted spoon and set aside.
2. Add the onion, green pepper and celery to the pan, put on the lid and cook for 5 mins, stirring occasionally until softened a little. Stir in the garlic, spices, thyme and bay leaf and cook for 1 min until fragrant. Return the chicken and any juices to the pan with the flour, stirring to coat everything. Pour in the tomatoes and stock, and bring to the boil, cook for 5 mins, then add the okra and half the sage. Turn down to a simmer, put on the lid and cook for 10 mins. Then season and serve, scattering the rest of the sage over.

Summer Veggie soup

Serves 2

- 1 tablespoon olive oil
- 1 leeks, finely sliced
- 1 celery sticks, finely chopped
- 2 courgettes, quartered lengthways then sliced
- 2 garlic cloves, finely chopped
- ½ vegetable stock
- 100grams asparagus, woody ends removed, chopped
- 50grams peas, fresh or frozen
- 100grams broad beans
- small bunch basil, most chopped

Method

1. Heat the oil in a large saucepan, add the leeks and celery, and cook for 8 mins until soft.
2. Add the courgettes and garlic. Cook gently for 5 mins more.
3. Pour in the stock and simmer, covered, for 10 mins.
4. Add the asparagus, peas and broad beans, and cook for a further 4 mins, until just cooked through.
5. Stir in the chopped basil and season well. Scatter with basil leaves and serve.

Steak with chimichurri sauce

Serves 2

- small bunch parsley, roughly chopped
- ½ teaspoon oregano, fresh or dried
- 2 garlic cloves
- 1 shallot, chopped
- ½ teaspoon chilli flakes
- 2½ tablespoon olive oil
- juice ½ lemon
- 2 teaspoon red wine vinegar
- 2 x 125gram rib-eye or sirloin steaks
- fries and salad, to serve

Method

1. To make the chimichurri, blitz the parsley, oregano, garlic, shallot and chilli flakes in a food processor or chop very finely by hand.
2. Add 2 tablespoon of the olive oil, the lemon juice, vinegar and some seasoning, and pulse to combine everything to a saucy consistency.
3. Rub the remaining oil and a little seasoning into the steaks.
4. Heat a griddle or frying pan and cook the steaks for 2-3 mins on each side or until done to your liking.
5. Rest for a few mins, then spoon over the sauce.
6. Serve with fries and salad.

Griddled chicken and corn cob salad

Serves 2

- 2 small skinless chicken breasts
- 1 garlic cloves, crushed
- ½ tablespoon paprika
- Juice 1/2 lemon
- 2 tablespoon olive oil
- 2 corn cobs
- 2 Little Gem lettuces, quartered lengthways
- Handful of watercress
- ½ cucumber, diced

Method

1. Cut the chicken breasts in half lengthways so you are left with 4 chicken strips.
2. Mix the garlic, paprika, lemon juice and 1 tablespoon oil with some seasoning and toss with the chicken.
3. Leave to marinate for at least 15 mins.
4. Heat a griddle pan and brush with half the remaining oil and cook the chicken for 3-4 mins each side until cooked through.
5. Brush over the remaining oil and griddle the corn cobs, turning to cook evenly, for about 5 mins or until lightly charred. Remove and cut off the kernels.
6. Mix the lettuce and cucumber, top with the corn and chicken, and drizzle over your choice of dressing.

Smoked salmon & avocado

Serves 2

- 2 ripe avocados
- 1 lemon, juice only
- 250g pack smoked salmon
- small handful tarragon, leaves only, chopped
- 4 tablespoon crème fraîche
- 1 tablespoon caper, drained

Method

1. Stone and peel the avocados, cut into chunks and toss in half the lemon juice.
2. Twist and fold the smoked salmon pieces onto serving plates, then scatter with the avocado.
3. Cover and chill for up to 1 hr until ready to serve.
4. Mix together the tarragon, crème fraîche and remaining lemon juice. Drizzle over the salmon, scatter with the capers and serve straight away.
5. Add some good quality bread to make this a real treat

Dishes under 400 cals

Moussaka light!

Serves 2

- 1 large onion
- 2 garlic cloves
- 300grams extra-lean lamb mince
- 1 teaspoon olive oil
- 2 courgettes
- 1 large aubergine
- 2 teaspoon dried oregano
- 1 carton or tin of chopped tomatoes with garlic and herbs
- 1 lamb or beef stock cube
- 200grams low-fat Greek yogurt
- 75grams feta cheese

Method

1. Preheat the oven to 190
2. Fry off the onions and garlic in a little oil and add the mince.
3. When the mince has browned add the chopped courgettes.
4. In a separate pan fry the sliced aubergine to brown lightly in the oil then set aside.
5. Add the tomatoes and half the oregano to the meat mixture.
6. Add the stock cube and season to taste with black pepper.
7. Spoon the meat mix into an oven proof dish and top with the aubergine slices.
8. Mix the crumbled feta, the rest of the oregano and the yoghurt and spoon over the aubergine to cover as evenly as possible.
9. Bake in the oven for 15 to 20 minutes.
10. Serve with a nice Greek salad on the side

Thai chicken parcels

Serves 2

- 2 skinless chicken breasts
- small pack coriander
- 1 pak choi
- 175g sugar snap peas
- 1 teaspoon fish sauce
- 1 teaspoon soy sauce
- 2 tablespoon rice vinegar
- 2 tablespoon sweet chilli sauce
- zest and juice 1 lime
- 1 tablespoon Thai green curry paste
- 100grams basmati rice

Method

1. Heat oven to 220C/200C fan/gas 7.
2. Heat a non-stick frying pan over a high heat and cook the chicken breasts for 4-5 mins on each side until browned.
3. Lay a large piece of baking parchment on a baking tray; add half the coriander, the pak choi and sugar snap peas.
4. Place the chicken breasts on top. Combine the fish and soy sauce, rice vinegar, sweet chilli, lime zest and juice, and curry paste, and pour over the chicken and veggies, then cover with another piece of parchment.
5. Fold up each edge to form a parcel and cook for 12-15 mins.
6. Meanwhile, cook the rice following pack instructions.
7. Remove the parcel from the oven, leave to sit for 1-2 mins, then cut open and add the rest of the coriander.

Ham and lentil salad with carrot

Serves 2

- 250grams ham chopped small or shredded
- 400grams can lentils
- 2 carrots – shredded or grated
- 4 celery sticks chopped small
- A medium bunch of parsley

For the dressing

- 2 tablespoon of olive oil
- 2 tablespoon of red wine vinegar
- 1 tablespoon of water
- ½ teaspoon of stevia
- 1 teaspoon of wholegrain mustard
- Black pepper and salt to taste

Method
1. Mix the salad ingredients in a bowl.
2. Whisk together the ingredients for the dressing.
3. Pour over the salad and give it a good mix up.
4. Serve

Turkey Nacho Bake
Serves 2

- 1 large onion
- 1 garlic clove
- 1 tablespoon olive oil, plus a little extra if needed
- 1 teaspoon ground cumin
- 250grams turkey mince
- 2-3 fresh chillies finely chopped
- 200grams tinned chopped tomatoes
- 200grams kidney beans
- 2 corn tortillas, cut into triangles
- small handful grated cheese – mozzarella is good
- 5 cherry tomatoes
- Half a red or green pepper
- 125ml water

Method

1. Preheat the oven to 190 degrees
2. Fry off the onions and garlic in the oil until soft.
3. Add the chopped chillies and cook for another minute
4. Add the cumin and cook for 1 minute more.
5. Stir in the mince and add a bit more oil, if required.
6. Cook for 4-6 mins, stirring occasionally, until the mince is browned.
7. Stir in the tomatoes and the water and simmer for 5 mins.
8. Mix in the beans and cook for a few mins more until thick piping hot and the mince is cooked.
9. Transfer to an oven proof dish
10. Scatter the tortilla triangles randomly on top.
11. Sprinkle the cheese and put in the oven for about ten minutes or until the cheese has fully melted
12. Chop the cherry tomatoes and pepper and mix together with a little salt and pepper to make a crunchy salsa.
13. When you remove the nacho bake from the oven dollop the salsa on the top and serve.

Chicken and kale stir-fry

Serves 2

- 2 chicken breasts sliced long and thin
- 1 garlic clove
- ½ Onion
- 100grams shiratake or vermicelli rice noodles
- 100grams shredded kale
- 2 teaspoon sesame oil
- 1 or 2 chillies (optional)
- 1 spring onion chopped small
- 5 or 6 mushrooms – oyster or shitake if you like but standard will be fine
- ½ and inch fresh grated ginger
- 1 red pepper sliced long and thin
- 3 courgettes cut into matchsticks
- 1 tablespoon light soy sauce
- 2 tablespoon rice wine or white wine vinegar

Method

1. Cook the noodles then drain and set aside or for shiratake noodles rinse and drain.
2. Wilt the kale in a pan with a little water – you still want it to have some texture – about one or two minutes should do the trick. Drain and set aside
3. In a wok or stir fry pan brown the chicken then remove and set aside.
4. In the same wok, adding a little more sesame oil if required, brown the onion and garlic.
5. Add the mushrooms, pepper, chillies, ginger, courgettes and fry for a few minutes
6. Add the chicken and kale and fry until the chicken is cooked through
7. Add the noodles. Give it a good stir to integrate the noodles fully into the dish

8. Tip in the soy sauce and rice wine and a little water if needed and stir well to coat all the ingredients.
9. Serve and enjoy

You could replace the chicken with prawns – it still tastes great. Or you can have chicken and prawns...

Smoked mackerel pasta

Serves 2

- 150grams slim pasta shapes rinsed and drained – you can use wholemeal pasta if you have not been converted to slim pasta yet ☺
- ½ onion
- 1 garlic clove
- 2 teaspoons olive oil
- 1 red pepper finely diced
- Juice and zest of 1 lemon
- 200grams smoked mackerel fillets – remove the skin
- 140grams half-fat crème fraîche or light cream cheese
- Small bunch of fresh parsley – chopped

Method

1. Cook the pasta, drain and set aside.
2. Brown the onion and garlic in the oil for a minute.
3. Add half the finely diced pepper
4. Add a little water to stop anything sticking.
5. Add the drained pasta and mix it all up.
6. Flake the smoked mackerel into the mixture
7. Add the lemon juice and loads of black pepper
8. Add the crème fresh and reduce the heat
9. Remove from heat
10. Serve sprinkled with the parsley and more black pepper

Chinese chilli beef

Serves 2

- 250grams lean beef, such as sirloin steak, trimmed of any excess fat
- ½ red pepper
- 4 spring onions
- 85grams tender stem broccoli
- 100grams pak choi
- 3 tablespoon fresh orange juice
- 1 teaspoon rice wine vinegar or white wine vinegar
- 2 teaspoon dark soy sauce
- 1 teaspoon hot chilli sauce
- 1 medium egg white
- ½ teaspoon five-spice powder
- 1 tablespoon cornflour
- 1½ teaspoon self-raising flour
- 2 tablespoon sesame oil
- 2 garlic cloves, finely chopped
- 2 teaspoon grated root ginger
- ¼ teaspoon chilli flakes,

Method

1. Put the meat in the freezer 25-30 mins before you plan to start cooking. This makes it easier to slice really thinly.
2. Slice the red pepper, spring onions, pak choi and broccoli long and thin.
3. Mix together the orange juice, vinegar, soy sauce and chilli sauce.
4. Slice the beef into very thin strips.
5. Beat the egg white with a fork to make it slightly frothy then add the five-spice powder, cornflour, flour and plenty of black pepper.
6. Add the beef strips to this mixture to coat them evenly

7. Stir fry the beef in one tablespoon of sesame oil for 3-4 minutes until browned. Remove and set aside
8. Add the remaining oil to the wok and stir fry the garlic and onions for a minute then add all remaining veggies and chilli and stir fry for another three or four minutes.
9. Add the beef back to the pan and stir for another minute.
10. Add the juice and soy mixture and bring to a bubble .(add a bit of extra water at this point if it seems too dry)
11. Serve piping hot.

Brown butter sole

Serves 2

- 1 teaspoon sunflower oil
- 50grams butter
- 4 lemon sole fillets
- 200grams frozen peas
- 100grams mussels, washed and de-bearded
- 2 tablespoon of dry cider
- Juice of ½ lemon
- Rocket and watercress to serve

Method

1. Heat the oil and butter in a deep frying pan until foaming.
2. Add the fish fillets and cook for 3-4 mins.
3. Carefully turn over and baste with the butter, which should be brown but not burned.
4. Increase the heat and add the peas, mussels, cider, lemon juice and loads of black pepper
5. Cover with a lid and cook for another 3-4 mins until the mussels have opened – discard any that remain closed.
6. Serve on a bed of rocket and watercress with lemon wedges on the side.
7. Or stick it on a bed of brown or wild rice.

Crab and Prawn cocktail (tribute to the 80's)

Serves 2

- ½ small fennel bulb, very finely sliced
- Juice ½ lemon
- 2 avocados
- Small bunch dill
- 1 Baby Gem lettuce
- 125grams cooked crabmeat
- 125grams cooked prawns
- lemon wedges, to serve

For the cocktail sauce

- 2 tablespoon mayonnaise
- 1 tablespoon ketchup
- A dash of Worcestershire sauce
- 2 drops Tabasco sauce
- zest ½ lemon
- large pinch of paprika and a little to decorate
- ½ red chilli

Method

1. Put the fennel in a large bowl of ice-cold water with a squeeze of lemon juice. After half an hour it will be very crisp.
2. Skin and dice the avocados but put them aside in a bowl with the avocado stone – this stops the avocado flesh going brown.
3. Whisk together all the ingredients for the cocktail sauce in a bowl with seasoning. Put in the fridge to chill.
4. Drain the fennel and toss with the remaining lemon juice, dill and loads of black pepper. Layer the lettuce, avocado, fennel, prawns and crab in two glass dishes layering until finishing with the cocktail sauce.
5. Sprinkle a pinch of paprika and serve.

Dishes under 500 calories

Asparagus and tuna salad

Serves 2

- 8 baby new potatoes
- 2 medium eggs
- 125gram pack asparagus
- 185gram can tuna, drained and flaked into very large chunks
- small handful small black olives, halved
- 1 romaine lettuce, leaves torn into chunks

For the dressing

- 1 shallot, finely chopped
- 1 teaspoon English mustard powder
- 2 tablespoon white wine vinegar
- 1 tablespoon extra-virgin olive oil, or use the oil from the tuna can (if bought in oil)
- ½ teaspoon of stevia

Method

1. Boil the potatoes for 8-12 mins until tender.
2. Drain and cool.
3. Put the eggs in a pan of cold water and bring to the boil
4. When the water boils add the asparagus for 2 mins.
5. Drain well and rinse everything under cold water to cool.
6. When the eggs are cool – shell them
7. Put all the dressing ingredients in a bowl with a tablespoon of water and mix well or whisk.
8. Mix all the salad ingredients together and add the dressing
9. Serve!

Rosemary roast chicken thighs, new potatoes, asparagus & garlic

Serves 2

- 350grams new potatoes – cut in half
- 250grams asparagus tips
- 1 whole garlic bulb
- 1 tablespoon olive oil
- 1 lemon
- 1 small bunch of rosemary
- 4 chicken thighs

Method

1. Heat oven to 200C.
2. Arrange the potatoes, asparagus, garlic cloves, oil and lots of seasoning in a large roasting dish.
3. Squeeze over all the lemon juice then chop up the lemon skin into chunks and add to the dish.
4. Mix it all up, cover with foil and roast for about 15 mins.
5. Remove the foil and add the rosemary.
6. Season the chicken thighs and arrange evenly in the dish.
7. Roast for another 25-30 mins until the potatoes are tender, and the chicken is crisp and cooked through.
8. Enjoy

Chilli prawn noodles

Serves 2

- 150grams medium egg noodles or up to two packets of rinsed drained shiratake noodles
- 1 tablespoon sesame oil
- 1 tablespoon groundnut oil
- 8 spring onions thinly sliced lengthways
- 300gram bag bean sprouts
- 4 garlic cloves
- 1 red chilli
- ½ inch of grated ginger root
- 300grams raw peeled tiger prawns
- 1 tablespoon dark soy sauce

Method

1. Cook the noodles following pack instructions,
2. Toss with 1 teaspoon of the sesame oil.
3. Heat 2 teaspoon of the groundnut oil in a non-stick wok.
4. Stir-fry the spring onions and the bean sprouts for a couple of mins until tender.
5. Add the noodles and warm through.
6. Stir through the remaining sesame oil and tip out of the wok onto a preheated serving dish.
7. Carefully wipe out the wok and add the remaining groundnut oil.
8. Add the garlic, ginger and chilli, and cook for about half a minute
9. Add the prawns and stir-fry until they are pink.
10. Stir in soy and cook until prawns are cooked through.
11. Serve on the noodles

Griddled chicken with Greek quinoa

Serves 2

- 130grams quinoa
- 25grams butter
- 1 red chilli chopped small
- 1 garlic clove – crushed and chopped
- 200grams chicken mini fillets
- 1 tablespoon olive oil
- 150grams cherry tomatoes quartered
- 20 pitted black kalamata olives
- ½ finely sliced red onion
- 50grams feta cheese, crumbled
- A handful of mint and a handful of parsley, chopped
- juice and zest ½ lemon

Method

1. Cook the quinoa following the pack instructions then rinse in cold water and drain thoroughly.
2. Make a paste with the butter, chilli and garlic.
3. Mix the chicken fillets in 2 teaspoon of the olive oil with some low salt and black pepper.
4. Cook on a hot griddle pan or in a 'health grill' and cook for 3-4 mins each side or until cooked through.
5. Transfer to a plate and smooth on the garlic and chilli paste and put to one side to melt.
6. Put the tomatoes, olives, onion, feta mint, parsley and quinoa into a salad bowl.
7. Stir through the remaining olive oil, lemon juice and zest, and add some low salt and black pepper to taste
8. Serve the chicken fillets on the salad and make sure to rescue any melted butter paste and add to the dish

Incredibly healthy soups

No calorie values added to this lot – just lots of healthy ingredients. Some our more calorific than others – just categorising them as low, medium and high. You are not dieting so just giving you a rough idea out of interest.....

Spinach soup (low)

- Enough olive oil to brown the onion, leek, mushrooms, potato, celery and garlic
- 1 onion
- 1 garlic clove
- 1 leek
- 1 small potato
- 5 or 6 standard mushrooms
- 1 litre of vegetable stock made as per instruction on cube.
- 1 bag of spinach
- Black pepper to taste

Method

1. Heat the oil in a large saucepan.
2. Chop the onion, leek, mushrooms, garlic, celery and dice the potato then add to the pan
3. Stir and put on the lid. Turn the heat down and sweat for 10 minutes. Keep an eye that is not sticking and stir occasionally.
4. Pour in the stock and add the pepper and cook for 10 – 15
5. Add the spinach and cook until wilted.
6. Remove about 80% of the veggies and a little juice and pulse it in a jug (or other) blender – taking care not to over fill it and don't burn yourself on the steam!
7. Reintroduce the puree to the pan and stir in well.
8. Serve either as is or you could even swirl a little low fat crème fraiche in the top and sprinkle some more pepper for effect.

Asparagus soup (low)

- 25grams butter
- a little vegetable oil
- 350grams asparagus spears
- 5 or 6 standard mushrooms
- 2 onions
- 2 garlic cloves
- 1/4 a bag of spinach
- 750ml vegetable stock
- Fresh ground black pepper to taste

Method

1. Chop the onions and garlic well and brown in a pan with the oil and butter
2. Chop and add the asparagus spears – don't use the woody bits at the end though.
3. Add the spinach and the stock and cook until the spinach has wilted.
4. Remove about 80% of the veggies and some of the liquid Stir through the spinach, pour over the stock, bring to the boil, and then blitz with a hand blender.
5. Remove about 80% of the veggies and a little juice and pulse it in a jug (or other) blender – taking care not to over fill it and don't burn yourself on the steam!
6. Reintroduce the puree to the pan and stir in well.
7. Serve either as is or you could save a few of the asparagus tips from the blender to pop on top.

Bacon and Asparagus soup (medium)

For bacon and asparagus soup add a couple of hundred grams of cooking bacon at the onion frying stage and cook well through. Try to make sure you blend most of the bacon at blending stage – or you can choose not too if you want a meatier soup.

Salmon noodle soup (medium with normal noodles low with shiratake noodles)

- 1 teaspoon toasted sesame oil
- 2 salmon fillets
- 1 garlic clove
- ½ inch fresh ginger , grated
- 6 spring onions
- 150grams shiitake mushrooms
- 125grams baby corn
- 1 litre chicken or vegetable stock – made up as per cube instructions
- 2 teaspoons Thai red curry paste
- 100grams vermicelli style noodles or shiratake noodles
- Juice of 1 lime
- 1 tablespoon light soy sauce
- ½ a teaspoon stevia
- 6 coriander leaves

Method

1. Slice the mushrooms, 5 of the spring onions, garlic, baby corn and salmon.
2. In a saucepan or wok lightly stir fry the spring onions, garlic, mushrooms, ginger and corn in the oil.
3. Remove from heat and add the red curry paste and stir well.
4. Return to heat and add the stock, stevia and noodles and cook until the noodles are softened.
5. Add the salmon slices and cook for about three minutes until the salmon is cooked through.
6. Remove from the heat stir in the soy sauce and lime juice and serve sprinkled with coriander and the last spring onion, finely chopped.
7. This makes quite a big portion and could probably serve 3 or 4.

Italian veggie soup (medium with standard pasta low with shiratake / slim pasta)

- 100 grams of cooking bacon finely chopped
- 2 garlic cloves
- 1 onion
- 1 carrot
- 1 celery stalk
- 2 courgettes
- 1 tablespoon olive oil
- ½ teaspoon stevia
- 1 tablespoon of tomato purée
- 2 tablespoons mixed herbs
- 1 teaspoon red pesto
- 200grams of mixed beans (tinned but drained)
- 300grams of tinned chopped tomatoes
- 700mls vegetable stock – made up as per instructions
- 100grams small pasta shapes or slim pasta (find on the internet)
- 12 basil leaves
- Black pepper to taste

Method

1. Finely chop the bacon, onion, garlic, carrot, celery and courgettes and fry off in the oil until soft.
2. Remove from the heat and stir in the stevia, tomato puree, mixed herbs and red pesto, mixing it up well.
3. Add the beans, tinned tomatoes and stock and pasta and bring to the boil then simmer for 20 minutes for normal pasta, 10 minutes for slim pasta.
4. Sprinkle with basil leaves and black pepper to serve.

Thai noodle soup

- 2 teaspoons toasted sesame oil
- 1 onion chopped small
- 1 garlic clove chopped and crushed
- 1 litre chicken or vegetable stock made up as per instructions
- 2 tablespoons green or red Thai curry paste
- ½ inch grated fresh ginger
- 50 grams oyster mushrooms
- 1 teaspoon Thai fish sauce
- 1 red chilli, seeds removed, thinly sliced
- 1 medium pak choi
- 100grams carrots – slice these so thin they are almost grated
- 100grams sugar snap peas or mange tout
- 50grams cooked rice noodles or shiratake noodles and rinsed in cold water
- ½ lime

Method

1. Heat the oil and fry off the onion and garlic until softening
2. Add the chilli and mushrooms, add a little stock to stop sticking
3. Remove from heat and stir in the curry paste, ginger and fish sauce
4. Add the stock, carrot, peas, sliced pak choi and noodles.
5. Bring to the boil and simmer for ten minutes. Add more water if you want a lighter soup base.
6. Serve. You could throw on some finely sliced spring onion to make it look prettier.

Summer vegetable soup (low)

- 3 tablespoon olive oil
- 1 leek
- 1 red onion
- 2 courgettes
- 2 garlic cloves
- 1l vegetable stock made up as per instructions
- 250grams asparagus, tips and stems but not the woody bits
- 100grams frozen peas
- 200grams mange tout or sugar snap peas
- 15 basil leaves
- Black pepper

Method

1. Heat the oil in a large saucepan and fry off the onion and garlic.
2. Add the leeks and celery, and cook until soft.
3. Add the courgettes and cook gently for 4 or 5 minutes.
4. Pour in the stock and bring to the boil
5. Add the asparagus and peas, bring back to the boil and simmer for another 5 minutes or so
6. Season well.
7. Tear the basil leaves and scatter them to serve

Classic Cabbage Soup (very low)

- ½ a cabbage
- Teaspoon of olive oil
- 1 large onion
- 2 garlic cloves
- 4 celery stalks
- 4 large carrots
- 2 leeks
- 1 litre of vegetable stock – made up as per instructions
- Black pepper

Method

1. Chop everything
2. Fry off the onions and garlic
3. Add the rest of the vegetables and seasoning
4. Bring to the boil and simmer until the vegetables are soft
5. Remove about 80% of the veggies and a little juice and pulse it in a jug (or other) blender – taking care not to over fill it and don't burn yourself on the steam!
6. Reintroduce the puree to the pan and stir in well.
7. Serve

Tasty vegetable fat burner (very low)

This is knocked up from a huge variety of thermogenic and very healthy foods but feel free to add or remove anything to vary the recipe – it is more of a guide! This makes quite a big batch as I tend to freeze it and use it as a standby when I have the urge for something warm and comforting.

- 2 litres vegetable stock
- 4 onions
- 4 garlic cloves
- 1 green pepper
- 1 red pepper
- 3 or four chillies – to your taste
- ½ a cabbage
- 20 mushrooms
- 6 large carrots
- 6 courgettes
- 200grams broccoli
- 200grams spinach
- 200 grams asparagus
- A good handful of fresh parsley
- A good handful of fresh basil
- 3 tins or tubs of chopped tomatoes (any variety – use your favourite)
- 1 tablespoon oregano
- A bit more stock if you like a brothier texture

Method
1. Chop everything
2. Fry off the onions and garlic
3. Add the rest of the vegetables and seasoning
4. Bring to the boil and simmer until the vegetables are soft
5. Remove about 60% of the veggies and a little juice and pulse it in a jug (or other) blender – taking care not to over fill it and don't burn yourself on the steam! Add more stock if the texture is too thick for you.
6. Reintroduce the puree to the pan and stir in well. Serve.

The 'Bringing it all together for sustainable change' bit

So far we have looked at various weight maintenance techniques and associated nutritional requirements. Diets do not work for a sustainable period of time although the short term benefits of quick weight loss, if only to boost your confidence, are plainly visible.

If dieting worked effectively the diet industry would put itself out of business and whilst we seek quick fixes for weight issues that may have taken the best part of twenty or so years to form the diet industry will be happy to take our money for the next quick fix.

I hope that this is the last time you ever buy anything with the word 'diet' in it.

The methods in this book, the rules, the pep talk and a little bit of nutritional information should help you make those small changes that mean you NEVER HAVE TO DIET AGAIN.

Just eating only when you are hungry and being aware of your body's requirements can lead to that intelligent relationship with food and to the size and shape you know you can achieve and that you deserve with a minimum of effort in a way that is enjoyable and sustainable.

You now have the basic information and tools to finally get to your ideal weight and size

In a year from now you will be trimmer and feel healthier.

You may achieve your ideal in less time but even when you have sustained it for a year you can still listen to your body – ignore your inner critic and just keep going.

Persistence not perfection

Enjoy the new you.